Liz Earle's Nat

By the same author

Vital Oils (Vermilion)
Save Your Skin with Vital Oils (Vermilion)
Eat Yourself Beautiful (BBC Publications)

LIZ EARLE'S
NATURAL
BEAUTY

*A Practical Step-by-Step Guide
to Making Lotions, Balms, Tonics and Oils*

VERMILION
LONDON

Published in 1993 by Vermilion
an imprint of Ebury Press
Random House UK Ltd
20 Vauxhall Bridge Road
London SW1V 2SA

Catalogue record for this book is available from the
British Library.

ISBN 009 1777550

Typeset in Palatino by SX Composing Ltd, Rayleigh, Essex
Printed in England by Mackays of Chatham

For Paddy
facile princeps

ACKNOWLEDGEMENTS

I should like to thank all those who shared their valuable knowledge with me whilst researching and writing this book. In particular, I am grateful to Len and Shirley Price, and also to Geraldine Howard of Aromatherapy Associates for their aromatherapy expertise and information on essential oils. I must also thank my tireless researcher Annie Bawtree as well as the back-up team, who include Laura Hill, Isobel Hinman, Rosie Sandberg and last, but never least, my husband Paddy.

ABOUT THE AUTHOR

Liz Earle is a popular television presenter and best-selling author with a special interest in health and beauty. She has presented her own highly successful television series, *Beautywise* and *Eat Yourself Beautiful* on BBC 1 and has also appeared regularly on ITV's *This Morning* programme. An award-winning journalist, former health and beauty editor of *New Woman* magazine, and with her own column in *Country Living*, Liz has a wealth of specialist knowledge, and a compelling enthusiasm for promoting better health and dispelling many of our modern beauty myths.

Liz Earle lives in London and Gloucestershire with her husband Patrick and two children.

Contents

Introduction

Modern cosmetology is shrouded in technical mystery and yet the formulae for many of our health and beauty remedies today are based on traditional techniques that have been handed down over the generations. In fact, modern scientific research is now endorsing much of the folklore surrounding natural therapies that have been used for centuries. Making your own health and beauty preparations is fun and easy to follow. It can also save a great deal of money. Water and alcohol are the two most commonly used skincare ingredients, so why pay pounds for a product that contains only a few pence worth of ingredients? Because commercial products are required to have a shelf-life of many months, or even years, they are made with low levels of active ingredients and large quantities of chemical preservatives. By contrast, homemade remedies can contain much more useful amounts of active ingredients such as essential fatty acids, vitamins and enzymes. In addition, you may tailor many lotions and potions to suit your own individual needs and make many remedies for yourself, your family and friends.

The recipes in this book range from simple blends of massage oils to more detailed descriptions of making soap and skin cream, for the more adventurous. Effective treatments for skin problems such as acne, eczema, psoriasis and ageing skin are also included. You will also find practical background information on all the ingredients used and where you can obtain them. Unlike many shop-bought toiletries, your own products avoid animal testing and you can choose to buy cruelty-free ingredients. You can also re-cycle containers and cut down on the enormous amount of packaging waste produced by commercial manufacturers. With the help of this book you will be able to transform your kitchen into a beauty playground and fill your bathroom shelves with impressive treatments for your face, hair and entire body.

1
Natural Beauty in History

Natural beauty care has played an important part in history, since the earliest civilisations when mankind first used many of the plants and other elements provided by nature. The pioneers of natural beauty treatments were probably the cavemen living in the Mesolithic period, 10,000 BC, who applied grease and castor oil to soften the skin, and tattooed their bodies with plant dyes as protection from the sun. Recorded formulae for skin softening lotions date back to Biblical times, where women made lotions from olive oil and spices which were rubbed into sore feet to keep them smooth and supple. Scented barks and dried roots were finely ground to make talcum powders, and precious aromatic oils were often rubbed into the hair to keep it smelling sweet.

The first lipsticks were made in the Ancient city of Ur, near Babylon, some 5000 years ago. Next door in Egypt, Cleopatra relied on several hundreds of natural beauty remedies to maintain her legendary powers of seduction. Her fragrances literally changed the face of history and Mark Antony was said to have been intoxicated by the scent of rose and patchouli oils on her skin. Cleopatra's beauty routine included bathing in ass's milk, and applying face packs made from crushed sesame seeds and barley. Like most Egyptian women, she also favoured the use of henna and walnut oil to keep her hair dark and glossy, and used black kohl crayons made from powdered antimony (a type of metal) around her eyes to dramatic effect. Her shimmering blue and green eyeshadows were made from finely ground semi-precious stones such as lapis lazuli and malachite, which had a practical as well as cosmetic purpose as they shielded the skin from the sun's strong rays. Less appealing were Cleopatra's lipsticks and rouge which came from the deep red pigment of crushed carmine beetles and powdered ant's eggs.

The women of Thebes and those who lived alongside the Nile were reputed to be the most beautiful in the world, and they certainly made full use of the many natural paints and powders for their face, body and hair. Egyptian queens and noblewomen were buried with scores of alabaster jars filled with lotions and potions to use on every part of the body. A cosmetic chest was also included for the after-life and contained sticks of kohl to outline their eyes, beeswax mascara and mirrors made from highly polished copper set into carved ivory handles. Compared to other cultures of that time, the Egyptians were extremely vain and prided themselves on their appearance.

It is no coincidence that cosmetics were first developed by the Ancient Egyptians, and drawings depicting the extensive use of elaborate eye make-up have been found in tombs built as far back as 5000 BC. Surprisingly, remains of eye make-up found in the pyramids show that it was often made from fairly harsh substances, such as lead sulphide and charcoal. Reddish brown face paints contained special clays with a high iron content to give them their colour, and there was even a recipe for an anti-wrinkle remedy made from bullock's bile and ostrich eggs.

The Ancient Egyptians can probably take the credit for devising most of the earliest beauty preparations and they were especially fond of highly aromatic perfumes. Relics found in the pyramids include precious perfume flasks and essential oil carriers, placed there to keep their owners smelling sweet in the after-life. Aromatic oils were sold by Arab traders who travelled across the Middle East with precious cargoes of spices, frankincense and myrrh strapped to their camels. These were highly prized and were worth even more than gold. We can learn a great deal of useful information from the beauty recipes that have been handed down from years gone by. In addition to cosmetics and perfumes, the Ancient Egyptians were the first to develop soap, made from a natural cleanser called *saponin*, which is extracted from the soap-root or soapwort plant. They also added animal fats and fragrant oils to the soap formula and used them for household cleaning as well as bathing.

The Assyrians in the Middle East also put perfumed oils in their washing water and were scrupulous about personal hygiene. Body-smoothing products were popular, and skin scrubs first made their appearance around 1000 BC. These were made from powdered pumice stone and were used by Assyrian women to buff the body and keep the skin smooth. Before showering (which they did frequently), the Egyptians and Assyrians would rub themselves with handfuls of sand to clean the pores. Both the Assyrian men and women took great pride in their hair and it was always worn elaborately braided, oiled and perfumed. Tiny balls of perfumed wax were tucked close to the scalp so that during long banquets the fragrance would be released by body heat, and trickle down the neck to last throughout the evening. Men kept their beards trimmed like topiary into exotic shapes, and facial hair was such an important symbol of strength and power that Queen Matshrtpdont took to wearing a false gilded beard on ceremonial occasions.

Applying make-up for a night out obviously took a great deal of time, as is illustrated by the cosmetic box of Thuthu, the wife of a nobleman, which is kept in the British Museum. It contains the following necessities: sandals, elbow pads (for resting on, as putting on make-up was a lengthy process), pumice stones to smooth the skin and remove body hair, eye pencils of wood and ivory to apply powdered colour, a bronze dish for mixing colours and three pots of face cream.

The Ancient Greeks also knew a thing or two about cosmetics, although their mascara made from a mixture of gum and soot does seem a bit crude. Greek women painted their cheeks with herbal pastes made from crushed berries and seeds to give them a healthy-looking glow. They also developed a more dangerous habit of using white lead and mercury on their faces, to give the complexion a chalky appearance. Unbeknown to them, these heavy metals were absorbed through the skin and resulted in many untimely deaths – an unfortunate trend which continued down the ages.

The Greek physician Galen recognised the problem and wrote, 'women who often paint themselves with mercury, though they be very young, they presently turn old and withered and have wrinkled faces like an ape'. As well as being a first-class physician, Galen is also credited with the original recipe for cold cream, based on beeswax, olive oil and rosewater. He also remarked that garden snails, when finely ground, made an effective moisturiser, and the unfortunate creatures were used in beauty preparations for several centuries. Less unpleasant Greek customs included using natural henna to stain finger- and toenails red in much the same way as we paint ours with nail varnish today. They also made false eyebrows from dyed goat's hair, which they attached to the skin with natural gums and resins.

It was the Romans, however, who established many of our modern beauty habits. As the Roman Empire swept through Europe it left behind a legacy of daily bathing in communal baths scented with rosewater. The Romans also introduced the habit of regular shaving for men, with razors made from sharpened bronze. Rich noblemen and women continued to bathe in ass's milk and Nero's Queen Poppeia travelled with her own string of donkeys to provide the milk for her baths. Roman noblewomen also popularised the use of natural cosmetics in Britain by wearing kohl around their eyes, painting their cheeks with red paste made from beetle shells, and rubbing sweet-smelling aromatic oils into their hair.

One aspect of their appearance which took up a great deal of time, was the dyeing and dressing of their hair. The Romans used many different types of natural hair dyes, including one made from the mineral *quicklime*, which gave their hair a lustrous, reddish-gold tinge. Walnut oil made by steeping walnut shells in olive oil was also used to keep the hair dark brown when it began to turn grey. In Ancient Rome, blonde hair was initially considered to be a symbol of a prostitute, but with the arrival of the Scandinavian slave girls, noblewomen began to dye their own naturally dark hair lighter shades of blonde using a concentrated infusion of saffron flowers. Rosemary and juniper were the main ingredients in hair tonics reputed to prevent hair loss, and emollient skin soothers were made from saffron flowers and beeswax.

Pliny the Elder also records the use of many natural beauty ingredients, including quince cream from Cos, saffron from Rhodes and rosewater from Phaselis. He also notes the extensive use of *chypre* from Cyprus, a musky, long-lasting perfume. Many of these ingredients are still present in modern cosmetics, and can be used in several effective homemade remedies. Other natural ingredients that have not stood the test of time quite so well include crocodile dung which, believe it or not, was a popular Roman face pack.

When the Romans invaded Britain they were appalled to find that the native inhabitants did not believe in bathing and quickly set about building communal baths, some of which still exist in spa towns such as Bath. However, once they had departed Britain during the fourth century, the practice of regular bathing died out, except for the occasional cold water plunge undertaken as a penance. Despite this lack of routine cleanliness, women during the Middle Ages did continue to wear some form of make-up, although rouge was only worn by prostitutes. Noblewomen continued to use white lead on their faces; they plucked their eyebrows and stained their lips dark red with plant dyes. Natural skincare remedies were also popular and most noblewomen had their own favourite recipe for keeping the complexion smooth. To combat the destructive effects of wearing lead paste on the face, masks were made using ground asparagus roots and goat's milk, which were rubbed into the skin with pieces of warm bread. Elaborate braided hair styles were also popular and a kind of hair gel was made from a mixture of swallow droppings and lizard tallow. During the Crusades, knights returned home with all kinds of exotic preparations never before seen in Britain. Essential oils became popular as perfumes and were also used as antiseptics to ward off the plague. The technique of soap-making was also imported from Italy, although for centuries to come soap was mainly used for washing dishes and clothes, not bodies.

The next era to change the face of history was the Renaissance, a period of great learning and cultural development which saw many improvements in the world of natural beauty. Ladies in Venice, including Catherine de Medici, even established their own society for cosmetic testing and beauty training. However, their new-found knowledge did not stop them from continuing to use the destructive lead paint on their faces, neck and cleavage. One new invention was the introduction of the beauty spot, originally made from small circles of black velvet, which were used to hide blemishes, such as warts, pimples and pox scars.

The philosophy of personal hygiene was also gaining ground and the first commercial toothpowders appeared, usually made from a mixture of dried sage, nettles and powdered clay. In the 1500s, Venetian noblewomen would also dye their hair by applying lotions derived from saffron flowers or sulphur, and baking them on to their heads by sitting in the hot summer sun. Although the Europeans in general were still suspicious of regular bathing (they believed that it weakened the body) they used a great deal of perfume, presumably to mask the inevitably unpleasant smell of body odour. In 1508 one of the first European perfumeries was set up by monks of the Dominican Brotherhood in Florence. They produced many popular fragrances included rhubarb elixir and melissa water, and developed scented orris powder made from ground iris roots, which was used to perfume clothes and household linen.

Queen Elizabeth I imported many Italian and French fragrances, including scented kid gloves which were made in the hillside village of Grasse in the south of France. Life in Grasse originally revolved around the tannery industry, but perfume quickly became more popular than gloves and other leather goods, so the village turned into one of the leading fragrance centres in the world. Queen Elizabeth I was also one of Britain's most celebrated users of natural beauty preparations and her many portraits illustrate her passion for red wigs and painted skin.

Elizabethan ladies still used white lead face paint and toxic mercury sulphide for rouge. Horace Walpole later wrote of 'that pretty young woman, Lady Fortrose . . . at point of death, killed like Lady Coventry and others of white lead, of which nothing could break her.' Lady Coventry herself was only twenty-seven when she died from lead poisoning absorbed through her skin. The poisonous white lead was mixed with vinegar to form a paste called *ceruse*. The finest was thought to come from Venice and was very expensive. The less wealthy fared much better as they had to use cheaper, safer alternatives made from sulphur and borax. White lead made the hair fall out, and the extensive use of *ceruse* throughout the Elizabethan era explains the fashion for high foreheads, as hairlines were worn away. Another reason for hair loss was the use of the corrosive oil of vitriol (sulphuric acid) mixed with rhubarb juice as a hair tonic and lightener. Lipsticks were a somewhat safer blend of cochineal and beeswax, and finely ground mother-of-pearl became popular as an iridescent eyeshadow. Although bathing was not fashionable, the ladies of the court did take care to keep their complexions clean. The great Queen herself washed her face alternately in red wine and ass's milk, while others used rainwater or even their own urine.

Herbal infusions were also used to keep the skin clear, including fennel and eyebright water. On the rare occasions when their hair was cleaned, it was not washed but dry shampooed using finely powdered clays that were combed through to absorb the build-up of grease and dirt. Whisked egg whites were used to tighten and glaze the skin, and beauty spots remained a popular ploy for concealing blemishes. Freckles were frowned upon and one remedy for their removal calls for an infusion of elder leaves mixed with birch sap and brimstone (sulphur) to be applied to the skin by moonlight and removed in the morning with fresh butter. Bear's grease was a popular base for rouge and skin creams, and make-up pencils were made by mixing plaster of Paris with plant pigments to form sticks, which were dried in the sun.

During the reign of Charles I, the first British toiletry company set up shop in London. A young Mr Yardley is recorded as paying the monarch a large sum to gain the concession to manufacture soap for the whole of the capital. Unfortunately, the records of his activities were destroyed in the Great Fire of London, in 1666, but we do know that Yardley used lavender as the main perfume ingredient. From this time on, skincare remedies became increasingly refined, and ladies of the court of James II used moisturisers made from spices and vanilla pods infused in honey. However, the use of lead-based *ceruse* on the complexions continued, so the trend for high foreheads and an absence of eyebrows was still fashionable. Children had their brows covered in walnut oil to decrease hair growth and eyebrows were shaved and replaced with more delicate versions made from mouse skin. Balls of fine shaving soap also appeared for the men, who would have visited a cut-throat barber for their daily shave.

In 1786 an Act of Parliament was passed to tax cosmetics, and from this we can derive an accurate list of what was available at the time. The cosmetics listed include essences, powders, wash balls and pomades such as 'tincture of peach kernels', 'essence of bouquet' and 'carnation of lilies'. Make-up pigments included rouge, blanche, vegetable rouge (made from the safflower thistle) and serviette rouge (which was applied with a small cloth). There was also 'liquid bloom of roses', 'cold cream' and 'beautifying cream'.

By the time of the French Revolution in 1789 natural cosmetics, for both men and women of the Court, was the height of fashion. Elaborate powdered wigs, rouge and face powder were used extensively, with the men often wearing far more than the women. Although shampoo had by now been invented, it was common for courtiers to keep their natural hair short and unwashed while wearing a wig on top. These were often so large that several unfortunate noblewomen died from burns suffered when their headpieces brushed passed the candlelit chandeliers. As the wigs were made from a mass of wool and animal grease they were highly combustible and a huge fire risk. The wigs were also extremely expensive, and groups of children were employed to sit on the shoulders of a grown-up and snatch them from the heads of courtiers as they rode past in their open carriages. From this time onwards it became fashionable to appear pale and interesting, and women's fashions focused on flimsy muslin dresses which were both diaphanous and daring. Sometimes they were even dampened to make them cling, often resulting in bronchitis and pneumonia for the unfortunate wearer.

However, as the Empress Josephine had an olive complexion (she was brought up in the West Indies), she continued to make herbal rouge an essential fashion accessory into the 1800s. One of the first beauty boutiques to supply the Parisian courtiers was opened in 1828 by Pierre Guerlain, founder of the famous French fragrance house. His shop was in the ground floor of the Hotel Maurice, in the Rue de Rivoli, where the dining room stands today. The many fragrant blends he created for the French Court included such patriotic perfumes as 'Bouquet Napoleon', 'Parfum de France' and 'Eau Imperial' (which is still available today). French noblewomen have a tradition of setting many beauty trends and Empress Eugenie, the beautiful wife of Napoleon III, was among the first to wear and popularise mascara made from waxes and natural plant pigments.

Over the centuries, herbalism and the study of plants had developed into an important medical science. One of the first to document the medicinal and beautifying properties of herbs was Master-Surgeon John Gerard, who was an enthusiastic botanist as well as a respected physician. One of his great medical advances was to identify the herb called scurvy-grass (*Cochlearia officinalis*) which is rich in Vitamin C and an effective cure for scurvy. According to Gerard, the plant grew alongside the banks of the river Thames and along stretches of Southern coastline – the very places where it was needed by the thousands of sailors who died from Vitamin C deficiency. In 1590, Gerard wrote a guide to herbalism which became a household bible throughout the country. Just like a well-thumbed cookery book today, Gerard's work was referred to almost daily for homemade herbal health and beauty recipes.

Probably the best-known English herbalist was Nicholas Culpeper. Born in 1616 the son of a Surrey rector, Culpeper studied Latin and medicine at Cambridge and might have gone on to become a doctor had his personal life not gone awry. After falling in love with a local girl, he borrowed £200 from his mother and ran away to get married. Culpeper arranged to meet his fiancée in Lewes, Sussex, but on the way there she was struck by lightning in a freak accident and killed. The distraught Culpeper abandoned his studies until eventually his grandfather set him up as an apprentice in a busy London apothecary. After his training, he turned his back on the lucrative medical world and opened a small shop in the deprived area of Spitalfields. Instead of prescribing expensive medicines he made 'cheap but wholesome medicines . . . not sending them to the East Indies for drugs, when they may fetch better out of their own gardens'. Culpeper believed that common herbs could be used to great effect in medicine and revived many of the teachings of the Ancient

Greek physicians such as Hippocrates and Galen. One of his favourite Biblical quotes was from Ecclesiastes: 'The Lord hath created Medicines out of the earth; and he that is wise will not abhor them'.

In 1649, Culpeper translated the *London Pharmacopoeia* into English from its original Latin – a move that outraged many doctors who wanted to keep their art secret. Culpeper went on to write his hugely popular book called *The Complete Herbal*, which was first published in the 1600s and has been reprinted throughout the centuries until the latest edition in 1979. Culpeper included many skincare remedies, including an infusion of vervain and broom stalks to cleanse the skin, oatmeal boiled with vinegar to treat spots and pimples, and wheat bread soaked in rosewater to soothe tired eyes. He also recommended woodbine ointment for sunburn, thistle juice for hair loss and rosemary oil for spots and scarred skin. In addition to his formulations, Culpeper also included astrological profiles for each plant as it was fashionable at the time even for doctors to consult the stars before prescribing remedies for their patients. For example, rosemary is under the sign of the Sun and is said to help cold disorders by warming and comforting the body, whereas vervain is a herb under the sign of Venus and so especially good for gynaecological problems.

Inspired by the herbalists, several beauty books were written during this time giving useful recipes and handy home hints. These were especially popular, for very few items of skincare or make-up could be bought over the counter. Although those living in big cities had access to a handful of up-market perfumeries, the rest of the country relied on travelling salesmen and homemade potions. One of the most popular books was *The Art of Beauty*, written in 1825 by an anonymous author who was quite likely to have been a doctor. The many recipes detailed include a hair strengthener made with two handfuls of hemp root, two handfuls of vine root and two handfuls of cabbage stalks. Nettle juice was also recommended to strengthen fine hair, or a more drastic action could be taken by shaving the head entirely and anointing the scalp with rosemary and dill oils.

Dental hygiene had at last become more popular and *The Art of Beauty* describes how to make your own toothbrush as follows: Collect two to three dozen fresh roots of marshmallow, each six ins. in length. Dry slowly and carefully in the shade so as not to shrivel before bruising the ends to make a brush. The tooth stick must then be soaked in an infusion made from the following ingredients: two ounces dragon's blood (the name given to a red resin from the trunk of the dragon tree), four ounces rectified spirit and half an ounce rose oil. Once the toothbrushes had dried they could then be used with a toothwash made from a bracing mixture of lemon juice, port and eau de cologne.

Less practical advice for ladies from *The Art of Beauty* includes erasing wrinkles by becoming overweight, applying powdered mint to reduce a large bosom, and using belladonna juice from the deadly nightshade plant to enlarge the pupils of the eyes. The author also advises us not to put stays on children and to avoid tight corsets when pregnant. But the doctrine for 'beauty training' makes modern health farms look like a holiday camp. Regency ladies were advised to observe the following regime:

Rise at six a.m. (or five a.m. but not sooner). Briskly walk two to three miles examining the flora, fauna and clouds as you go. On returning home, change if you have perspired and dry your feet. Have all your skin, particuarly that of the stomach, well rubbed with a cloth or flesh brush. Wash hands and face in cold water.

Breakfast Plain biscuit (not bread), broiled underdone beefsteak or mutton chop with no fat, and half a pint mild ale.

Morning occupation Out of doors, walk, garden, romp etc.

Dinner at two p.m. As breakfast (no vegetables, boiled meat, fruit, sweets or pastry) plus the occasional mealy potato or boiled rice.

Afternoon occupation Out of doors, walk, garden, romp etc.

Supper at seven p.m. Much as breakfast and dinner.

Evening At least an hour's active exercise.

Bedtime Ten p.m. or earlier. Bathe feet in tepid water and rub as before.

The only advantages of this Spartan routine were to put colour back into the cheeks and to acknowledge the need to wash.

A fellow advocate of regular bathing at this time was the Prince Regent, later George IV, who installed an extensive bathroom at his Brighton Pavilion. Exclusively for men, the large tub was filled with a mixture of hot water and milk with herbs such as flax seeds (linseeds) to soften the skin. With the arrival of Queen Victoria on the throne came a new fervour for bathing throughout the country. However, there were no skin creams or cosmetics in polite society and only a dab of eau de cologne was deemed respectable. When out of doors complexions were always protected by green veils (white netting encouraged the sun's rays) and by wearing bonnets with big brims. Inside, the face was shielded from the glare of the fire by pole screens.

Some women obviously rebelled against this puritanical regime and in 1909 a Mrs and a Miss Earle (no relation!) went to Paris as beauticians, where they set up the English Institute of Beauty in the Rue St Honoré. Their cosmetic preparations included face powder made from finely ground rice flour, tinted with carmine and scented with rose oil. Powdered chalk and zinc oxide were introduced to whiten the skin, although white lead and mercury continued to be included in many face powders. Other minerals used in cosmetics at this time included lead filings and iron dust, which were boiled in vinegar and used to dye the eyebrows. Moisturisers were made from a mixture of glycerine, barley flour and honey, and cold cream was much the same as Galen's original Greek recipe.

While the Victorians thoroughly disapproved of vanity they viewed cleanliness as being next to godliness. Soap became more widely available for those who could afford to buy it, although it was not until the middle of the century that most houses were built with indoor bathrooms. Until then, baths were taken in a tin tub in front of the sitting-room fire. At this time, soap was readily available but was sold in long anonymous bars which had to be sliced on the grocer's counter.

The first commercial soap was produced in 1884 by a Lancashire grocer called William Hesketh Lever. He had the brainwave of pre-cutting manufactured bars of soap, and stamping them with the brand name Sunlight. Demand soon overtook production and in 1888 William Lever bought a stretch of Mersey marshland and put Port Sunlight on the map of Britain. Although it sounds obvious today, William Lever's idea to give a bar of household soap a good name, wrap it properly and sell it energetically was an entirely new marketing concept. From these humble beginnings rose many other well-known soap brands, such as 'Lux', 'Lifebuoy' and 'Shield' – and so the mighty multi-national detergent giant Lever Brothers was born. Even today, this company remains the largest supplier of soaps in the world.

Queen Victoria herself may have disapproved, but many other toiletry companies were founded during the Victorian era, including Coty and Cyclax. Yardley continued to go from strength to strength, and had branched out from cakes of lavender soap into a skincare range that included 'Milady Powders', 'Lavender Vanishing Cream' and 'Lavender Cold Cream'. Ideas for marketing and advertising began to emerge and Yardley adopted as its trademark an illustration of a group of flower sellers, with the girls holding primroses and not bunches of lavender.

At the end of the Victorian era a more relaxed attitude was taken to make-up, and publications such as *Vogue* and *The Queen* magazine started to support the infant cosmetic industry. Sarah Bernhardt was reported to add half a pound of marshmallow flowers and four pounds of bran to her baths each day. She also endorsed 'Bernhardt Wrinkle Eradicator', a cream made from aluminium paste, almond milk and rosewater.

Across the Channel, Helena Rubinstein had left her native Poland and opened a salon in Paris where she sold a moisturiser called 'Creme Valaze'. Helena was the eldest of eight sisters renowned for their beautiful complexions, and her skin cream – made by a pair of Polish chemists – became the cornerstone of what would become her cosmetic empire. Another Parisian contemporary of Helene Rubinstein was M. Coty, a perfumier who was struggling to get his fragrances accepted in Paris. His big break came, quite literally, in 1903 when he tried unsuccessfully to get one of the larger shops to stock his scent. The manager refused even to open the bottle, but on the way out M. Coty smashed the bottle on the floor, the customers liked what they smelt and he was in business.

America was also busy building its own cosmetic empires and one of the first was established by Charles Meyer in 1860. A German wigmaker, Mr Meyer set up a small shop on Broadway selling Leichner's theatrical make-up, the first grease paint make in the USA. But a grease-based make-up requires something to remove it with, and for this, 'Pond's

Extract' was used – first distributed in 1846 by Theron T. Pond and later to become famous as 'Pond's Cold Cream' or 'Vanishing Cream'. At the turn of the century it was also discovered that zinc oxide made a good face powder – which did not discolour or harm the skin – and in Hollywood, yet another immigrant wigmaker called Max Factor was making a name for himself designing make-up for the stars of the silent screen.

Early movie-making was extremely primitive and stars of the black and white movies, like Clara Bow, had to paint their faces with blue and brown panstick before their features could be seen clearly on the screen. Max Factor's Panchromatic make-up became so important to the stars of that age that it even won him an Academy Award in 1928. As moviemaking progressed, Max Factor discovered a demand for coloured pansticks and foundations for the colour 'talkies' and went on to invent a flesh-tinted make-up stick called 'Erase', which sold over 10 million units in its first year. His competitors included Elizabeth Arden, who had developed a range of make-up and skincare based on natural ingredients. Elizabeth Arden herself was born in Canada and christened Florence Nightingale Graham – her name initially leading her to train as a nurse. However, she was so impressed by the well-groomed American women she came across that she retrained in a beauty salon. When she opened her own salon in New York's Fifth Avenue she searched for a more suitable name and was inspired by the book she was reading at the time called *Elizabeth and Her German Garden*, which contained verses from Tennyson's poem 'Enoch Arden'.

Dorothy Gray was another American who opened a rival salon on Fifth Avenue, where she specialised in treatments for sensitive skins. Her massage treatments – which she carried out – were so popular that she insured her hands for a record US$100,000. Although Dorothy Gray's original skincare line has now disappeared, her name still appears on a range of toiletries made closer to home in Eastbourne, Sussex.

A longer-lived success story is that of Estée Lauder, one of the few women to become a legend in her own lifetime. Estée Lauder started up her business in 1946 by selling just four skincare products to the smart Saks Fifth Avenue department store in New York. From this humble beginning she founded the now world-famous cosmetic company which she still tightly controls.

Back in Britain, however, the rigours of war-time rationing meant that there was very little in the way of glamorous make-up or beauty preparations. Women once again re-sorted to home remedies, including using gravy browning or strong tea to dye the legs in the absence of silk stockings. The restrictions on alcohol meant more concentrated perfumes and fewer eau de colognes were available, and the lack of fats, oils and glycerine resulted in skin creams being in short supply. Packaging was also a problem for many manu-facturers, with all the scrap metal being turned into munitions instead of make-up compacts. However, the beauty editor of *The Queen* magazine did find time to mention Max Factor's 'Pan Cake' make-up, recommending it 'particu-larly for women in the Forces or on other National work as it is very quick and easy to use and will stay on the skin for many hours . . . in six lovely shades from a pale flesh tint to a deep warm tan, in keeping with the colouring of the Woman's Service Uniforms.' A more important war-time purchaser of 'Pan Cake' was the Ministry of Defence, who ordered specially formulated shades to darken the faces of Commandos for night excursions.

After the war, developments in new cosmetics continued apace, and throughout the fifties and sixties, make-up and skincare moved further away from Mother Nature and in-creasingly into the realms of technology. The concept of anti-ageing creams that might actually turn back the clock was introduced, together with its often ridiculously outlan-dish claims. Yet despite the catchy slogans and youthful models with artfully re-touched skins, we have yet to en-counter a skin cream that can cope with crow's feet. In the last decade, the cosmetic and toiletry business has spent literally billions of dollars in search of the elusive elixir of youth that will wipe away all wrinkles. New ingredients have appeared on the scene such as bovine collagen (made from cow fat) which claimed to be able to plump up the skin and give it a youthful appearance. The only problem with this is that the collagen molecules are far too large to penetrate even the uppermost layers of skin cells.

In a further refinement of technology, new 'delivery systems' were invented to carry complex ingredients into the skin where they might target ageing skin cells. Microscopically small liposomes were developed to slip through the surface of the skin where, in theory, they could release their cargo of active ingredients to individual skin cells. These active ingredients include nutrients such as vitamins, essential fatty acids, fruit acids and natural sugars. Ironically, it has been the search for the most up-to-date and effective ingredients that has taken many cosmetic scientists back to nature's doorstep. Natural ingredients such as plant oils and herbal extracts are once again becoming increasingly popular as scientists begin to prove their legendary powers in the laboratory. Plant extracts such as chamomile have been found to heal damaged skin, avocado oil has been shown to regenerate ageing cells in mice, and Vitamins C and E are now known to be amongst the best anti-ageing ingredients of all times. This is good news for us, as consumers. In fact, there has never been a better moment to combine the knowledge that has been gathered by physicians, herbalists and beauticians over the last few thousand years and combine it with modern techniques to make the best natural beauty preparations for ourselves.

2
Getting Started

The recipes for making your own natural beauty products are remarkably simple. You do not need to be a cosmetic scientist or have a degree in biotechnology to produce naturally effective products in your own kitchen. All the recipes in the book have been tried and tested, but you may find some of the textures unusual. For example, the moisturising skin creams tend to be more concentrated than commercial lotions, as they have not been whipped with water and air to make them light. You may also find that some of the recipes vary according to the temperature, as ingredients such as coconut oil and cocoa butter are naturally harder in colder weather or if stored in a cool place.

Most of the ingredients I use are readily available from all good chemists, supermarkets, greengrocers and healthfood shops. To make life even easier, this chapter lists the basic ingredients you will come across in the book, together with a description of how each one can be used. This means that you look up the properties of a particular ingredient and adapt a recipe to suit your own skintype, or devise your own concoctions in the future. A large percentage of the ingredients are probably sitting in your kitchen or bathroom right now, and it is remarkable how many everyday items such as oatmeal and olive oil can be put to good use on the skin. Others, such as herbs or fruits, can be grown in the garden or on a window sill to provide a year-round source of fresh ingredients. These are listed in more detail in Chapter Three. If you have difficulty finding some of the more unusual ingredients, there is also a comprehensive list of stockists at the end of the book, as well as a glossary on page 161 to explain the more technical terms.

Useful equipment

Although there is little you need in the way of special equipment to start making your own beauty preparations, the following items will be helpful to have at hand. If you decide to make lots of your own recipes in the future, it might be worth keeping a set of utensils, such as spatulas, separate from the ones you use for cooking. This helps prevent the risk of cross-contamination of germs and odours, and means that your face cream will not end up smelling of onions.

Plastic measuring spoons to accurately measure tiny quantities
Set of small scales
Heat-proof jugs or small bowls
Enamel, stainless steel or Pyrex saucepan (not aluminium or cast iron, which can react with ingredients such as lemon juice)
Fine mesh sieve
Disposable coffee filters (to take tiny particles out of liquids)
Small funnel for decanting liquids
Rubber spatula or palette knife
Metal mixing spoons (avoid wooden spoons, which absorb ingredients such as essential oils)
Pipette (for measuring drop by drop, available from chemists)
Optional extras:
　　Blender or food processor
　　Pestle and mortar
The following are useful for packaging and storage:
　　Selection of bottles and jars, preferably made from glass so they can be sterilised and recycled

Sterilising fluid or tablets (from chemists)
Spray bottles (from chemists and department stores)
Paper towels (more hygienic than kitchen cloths for mopping up, etc.)
Sticky labels to name and date all items
Cardboard boxes for storing finished items in the cool and dark

Storage tips

Unlike commercial beauty products, the recipes in this book do not contain added chemicals to prolong their shelf-life artificially. You will not find common skincare chemicals such as ethyl or isopropyl alcohols, parabens and ammonium compounds or benzoic acid added to these natural remedies. However, steps must be taken to guard against bacterial or microbial spoilage and decomposition. Unfortunately, the basic oil and water mixture of many natural products is an excellent breeding ground for germs and a pot of cream is constantly exposed to new ones each time we dip our fingers into it. Products most susceptible to spoilage include those made with fresh ingredients such as fruits and vegetables, although even these will usually keep for several days in a cool fridge. The quantities given for the recipes in this book are therefore designed to make relatively small amounts to avoid spoilage and subsequent wastage. Products stored in the fridge should be kept separate from food, such as in a salad drawer or in a cardboard box on the top shelf.

Make a habit of labelling every item with its name and the date of making so you know when to discard it. If in doubt – throw it out! Most skin creams can be safely stored in the bathroom cupboard, but keep them out of direct sunlight, which will encourage rancidity. A small disc of greaseproof paper placed on the top of each jar of cream helps to keep the air out and prolong shelf-life.

Adding Vitamin E from capsules or from a few drops of wheatgerm oil also helps, as this nutrient acts as a natural preservative and prevents spoilage. Other natural preservatives include the antiseptic essential oils, notably lavender or menthol, which have been added to beauty preparations for this reason for thousands of years.

Hygiene hints

Bacterium love to breed in warm, moist conditions, so make life difficult for the bugs by keeping your equipment and preparation area as cool and dry as possible. All equipment, including final packing containers and lids, must be sterilised by dipping in sterilising fluid before using (alternatively, use a mild bleach solution and rinse well in boiled water). Whenever a recipe calls for water, only use filtered, boiled then cooled water, or distilled water, which is available from the chemist. Some varieties of bottled water may also be used, but choose reputable brands that have stringent quality controls and use those with low levels of minerals such as sodium (salt). Plain tap water contains many unwanted extras such as nitrates, chlorine, fluoride, traces of pesticides, etc., and should not be used at all. It sounds obvious, but always wash your hands before you start.

Allergy testing

Most natural skincare remedies are well-suited to those with sensitive skins as they do not contain the artificial colourants and fragrances that often lead to allergic reactions. Perfume contains as many as two hundred separate chemical ingredients, any one of which can trigger an adverse skin reaction. However, natural does not always equal safe and it is important to remember that even some completely natural substances can be dangerous if they are not handled with knowledge and care. Substances such as arsenic and lead are totally natural, yet we would not dream of using them on the skin. Likewise, many herbs and plant extracts have powerful effects that should not be under-estimated, and must be treated with respect. In the lists that follow you will find more detailed information on the safety of some of the stronger ingredients. Also, bear in mind that your own skin may not suit a particular ingredient or recipe. Although less likely to cause an allergic reaction than many chemical fragrances or preservatives, even basic natural ingredients such as lanolin or lemon juice can pose a problem for a few people. For this reason, it is wise to carry out a patch test whenever trying an ingredient or recipe for the first time.

How to do a patch test

Apply a small amount of the product or ingredient to be tested on an area of fine skin, such as the inner elbow. Cover with a sticking plaster and leave in place overnight. Should any unusual reaction, such as itching or redness, occur, bathe the affected area with a weak bicarbonate of soda solution and apply a soothing ointment such as calendula cream. Keep a record of the recipes you have tested and the ingredients which you know are suited to your skin. This will save time re-testing new products made with ingredients that you know are safe for your skintype.

Raw materials

The following ingredients can be found in chemists or health food shops:

Acetone

A harsh, colourless liquid that should be used with great care. It is highly flammable and is used as a thinner for paints and varnishes, including nail polish. It can be used sparingly as an inexpensive nail polish remover, but a small amount of almond oil should be added before use as it is extremely drying. Used in large amounts acetone can cause skin rashes, and inhaling its pungent fumes can also irritate your lungs. However, small quantities of neat acetone can be dabbed carefully on to spots and pimples as its drying action will remove any excess sebum or oil from the skin's surface.

Aloe Vera Juice

This succulent African plant looks like a spineless cactus and is reputed to have been used by Cleopatra as a skin cleanser. It is a member of the lily family and has fat, rubbery green leaves which produce a thick, clear gel when cut. Aloe vera juice is made from the plant's natural gel and has been analysed as being 99.5 per cent water. However, the remaining .5 per cent contains over twenty different amino acids and carbohydrates and many magical and mystical properties are credited to the plant's unusual juice. Aloe vera juice soothes and softens the skin and can help heal severe burns. Studies at the University of Pennsylvania Radiology Department have found that the juice of this plant is more effective in treating radiation burns than any other known product. As a result, the American army have stockpiled significant quantities to be used on troops in the event of a nuclear disaster. Aloe vera juice is available in bottles from healthfood shops and can be added to tonics and cleansers to soothe the skin.

Almond Oil

This colourless plant oil is extracted from the oil-enriched kernels of sweet, ripe almonds grown mainly in the Mediterranean. It is an important ingredient in moisturising soaps, creams and skin treatments and can even be used neat as a nourishing hand and nail massage oil. A refined form of almond oil is available from the chemist, and some supermarkets also sell a gourmet version of the oil that is suitable for skincare use.

Arnica Tincture

Made from the dried flowes of the arnica plant, arnica has many uses in skincare. It is an efficient skin soother and is especially useful for drawing out bruises or easing aches and sprains. Used for centuries by homeopathic doctors, tincture of arnica is one of our most effective remedies for sore, swollen skin, but should not be applied to scratches or open wounds (see *The Botanicals*, page 43).

Avocado Oil

This traditional beauty oil was first used by the tribeswomen of Mexico and Arizona where the avocado pear tree grows wild. The avocado itself is a highly unusual fruit as it takes two years to ripen and its flesh contains nearly fifty per cent plant oil. The natural oil is highly nutritious and is a good source of Vitamins A, B, D, E and lecithin. Although high in calories, the avocado does not contain any cholesterol and is a good source of the fatty acid linoleic acid, which strengthens the membranes surrounding skin cells. It also contains as yet unidentified substances that have been shown to help regenerate skin cells. Generally, the darker the avocado oil the better, as this means that it has undergone minimum processing and is likely to retain more of its natural nutrients. Avocado oil has a nutty smell and is one of the best oils for soothing dry, parched skins. It is available in either liquid form or capsules, which can be pierced with a pin and added to skin creams.

Balm of Gilead

This tincture is extracted from the buds of the poplar tree, common in Asia and North America. These reddish brown buds are coated with a sticky resin that is collected and made into Balm of Gilead. Its use as a skin-soothing ingredient and also as a pleasantly pungent perfume has been documented since Biblical times. Balm of Gilead contains a type of painkiller called *salicin* which is also found in aspirin and is used in medical herbalism as an antiseptic and stimulant, especially when treating coughs and colds. The tincture is also a mild circulatory stimulant and can be used in skin lotions to tone and strengthen the epidermis or upper layer of the skin, although it should not be used near the eyes or mouth.

Borax

This white powder consists of alkaline crystals and comes from a mineral that is mined in North and South America. It is a form of the trace mineral boron, which is used by the body to keep bones and teeth healthy and strong. Commonly used as a water softener, preservative and skin soother, borax also acts as an antiseptic, although it should not be used on broken skin. Borax has soothing properties and is used in many beauty products including soaps, shampoos, eye gels and moisturisers.

Calamine Lotion

This old-fashioned skin lotion is made from the *rhizome* or root of the sweet flag plant (*Acorus calamus*). Calamine lotion also contains zinc oxide, with five per cent iron oxide added to turn the liquid a pale pink colour. The liquid has drying and cooling properties and is useful for sore, sunburnt skin. It can also be found in astringent skin tonics and some facial washes.

Castor Oil

Extracted from the small, thorny castor bean plant that grows in India, Canada and North America, this thick oil is a colourless or yellow liquid which is pressed from the beans of the castor plant. These beans are poisonous, but the toxic protein *ricin* is left behind in the mulch after pressing. Purified castor oil is used in hairdressings such as brilliantine to give the hair a glossy shine, and in waxy cosmetics such as lipticks. It is a useful cosmetic ingredient as it leaves a shiny film on the surface of the hair and skin, and also acts as a waterproofing agent for barrier and nappy rash creams. Castor oil rarely causes a reaction on the skin and is even used in some eye-drop mixtures.

Cocoa Butter

This is the solid fat made from the roasted seeds of the cocoa tree. These seeds also give us chocolate and cocoa, and cocoa butter itself has a naturally sweet, chocolatey smell. The cocoa tree was first discovered in the sixteenth century by a Spanish explorer visiting the South American country of Mexico. He brought the cocoa bean back to Europe where it was processed into a sweet, chocolatey drink. It was not until the nineteenth century that the beauty benefits of the cocoa bean were fully realised. In 1828, the invention of the cocoa press made it possible to squeeze and filter the ground beans, extracting a liquid cocoa butter and leaving a dry low-fat cake of cocoa. This process signalled the start of the chocolate industry as we know it today and also introduced us to cocoa butter as a moisturiser. One of its most notable properties is that it melts at body temperature, and is therefore good for rubbing into the skin. Cocoa butter is a useful body moisturiser and also has the reputation for helping prevent stretchmarks (pregnant women in Tahiti traditionally rub lumps of solid cocoa butter over their stomachs to keep stretchmarks at bay).

Coconut Oil

This semi-solid plant oil looks more like a cream; it is so full of saturated fat it solidifies at room temperature. Coconut oil comes from the dried flesh of the coconut which contains around sixty-five per cent natural oil. It is often added to cosmetics and toiletries as it does not go rancid easily and is a good natural cleansing agent. It has low-lathering detergent properties and can be used to make shampoos and gentle washing-up liquids. Coconut oil is also commonly added to soaps and body lotions. It may also be used on its own as an effective dry skin moisturiser, or mixed with a few drops of sandalwood oil to make a fragrant hair shiner.

Evening Primrose Oil

The evening primrose is a tall, spiky plant with vivid yellow flowers that bloom in the evening, hence its name. It is not related to the common primrose but to the bay willow herb, and its oil comes from thousands of tiny, dark brown seeds. Although the origins of the evening primrose can be traced back by fossil remains to some 70,000 years ago, it is only recently that skincare scientists have been taking this unusual flower seriously. The secret to the plant's success is its oil which has a highly unusual fatty acid composition. All oils contain essential fatty acids which are good for the skin both internally and externally; however, evening primrose oil contains a type of essential fatty acid known as gamma linolenic acid, commonly shortened to GLA. Evening primrose oil contains about nine per cent pure GLA, which is an unusually large percentage.

The only other sources of GLA are blackcurrant seeds, borage oil and human breast milk. Borage oil itself is a richer source of GLA than evening primrose oil, but more difficult to find. GLA has been found to be helpful when taken in capsule form for treating hormonal problems such as PMS, symptoms of the menopause and for controlling eczema. Evening primrose oil can also be rubbed into patches of eczema to aid the healing process and may be added to moisturising creams to enrich them. Many skincare ranges now add evening primrose oil to their products; but, on the whole, they use such tiny quantities that their value on the skin is questionable. A more effective method is to make your own creams using higher quantities of this natural oil. The easiest way to obtain evening primrose oil is to pierce a capsule with a pin and squeeze out its contents. Alternatively, the oil is also available in a dropper bottle for more accurate measuring.

Fuller's Earth

This is sold in small packets and looks like powdered clay. In fact, Fuller's earth is mined from reclaimed areas of the seabed, where it is created from the remains of single-cell algae laid down over millions of years. It is so-called because fullers have used it for centuries to extract the natural grease or lanolin from sheep's wool. The fuller was an important member of the textile industry, whose job was to make the cloth heavier or more compact during manufacture by shrinking and beating or pressing. Fuller's earth itself is a highly absorbent cosmetic ingredient and works by drawing out dirt and embedded impurities from the skin. This makes it good for recipes such as deep-cleansing face and body packs. Fuller's earth is also a rich natural source of *silica*, an important mineral for maintaining skin strength and suppleness.

Glycerine

Most glycerine is extracted from animal fat, although some vegetable glycerine is becoming more widely available from herbal suppliers. The glycerine that is sold in chemists is made when animal fat or lard is heated industrially and a sticky, colourless liquid siphoned off. Glycerine mixes well with both water and alcohol and is an efficient skin softener. It is a *humectant*, which means that it attracts water. This makes it useful for attracting moisture from the atmosphere into the skin, but an excess can also draw out the skin's own natural water content and lead to dryness. It is used in making clear soaps and other skin soothers, such as moisturisers and aftershave balms.

Henna

This natural pigment comes from the henna plant, which is native to Egypt, the Middle East and India. Its first recorded reference is in the Bible in the Song of Solomon, where it is referred to as 'camphire'. Made from powdered leaves and stems of the shrub, henna is a natural hair and skin dye. The henna is mixed with water to form a paste to dye the hair various shades of red or brown. The drawback with using natural henna is that the results can be unpredictable and it should only be used after carrying out a patch test to establish the shade of the finished result.

Henna should be kept away from the eyes and should not be used to dye either eyelashes or eyebrows. Henna leaves are also used occasionally by herbalists for their astringent and anti-bacterial qualities.

Hydrogen Peroxide

This colourless liquid has powerful bleaching and antiseptic properties. It is commonly used in the cosmetic industry as a preservative. A three per cent solution can be bought from the chemist and used medicinally as an antiseptic and germicide. Useful for dabbing neat on to spots, pimples and boils, hydrogen peroxide should not be used on sensitive areas of mucous membrane such as the eyes, nose and mouth.

Jojoba Oil

Pronounced ho-ho-ba, this pale yellow oil is, in fact, a liquid wax that comes from the seeds of the evergreen jojoba plant grown mainly in Mexico. Traditionally used by the Aztecs and the Mexican Indians, jojoba oil is another of Mother Nature's beauty assets and remains an important ingredient in many modern scalp and skin lotions. Jojoba oil is unusual because it is the only wax that is naturally liquid at room temperature. It is very similar in chemical composition to sperm whale oil, called *spermaceti*, which was widely used in skincare creams until the early eighties. Jojoba oil also closely matches the skin's own oil, called *sebum*, and this makes it a good oil to use in facial treatments, especially for oily skins. Another benefit is that jojoba oil has a lengthy shelf-life and, unlike most other vegetable oils, does not spoil when left open to the air and sunlight.

Kaolin

Also known as China clay, kaolin originated from the Kao-ling hill in the Kiang-si province of Southeast China. Kaolin is a pure type of clay and can be used in beauty recipes instead of Fuller's earth. Kaolin is now mined in many parts of the world, notably Cornwall, China and Japan (where it is used to make their traditional chalky-white face powders). It is highly absorbent and attracts moisture; for this reason it is found in many talcum powders and deodorants. It is also used in the manufacture of porcelain and bone china, and in many remedies for diarrhoea such as kaolin and morphine. Kaolin is also an important ingredient of deep-cleansing face packs and abrasive tooth powders.

Lanolin

Chemically speaking, lanolin is a wax, not a fat, although it is often described as the natural fat found in sheep's wool – produced by the animal to provide an extra layer of insulation against harsh winters. Most fleeces contain around twenty per cent lanolin. Lanolin can be safely extracted after the sheep have been sheared, and does not involve killing the sheep. Lanolin is extracted either by dipping the fleece into alcohol to dissolve the fats present, or the fleece can be scrubbed in soap. As an ingredient, lanolin sinks into the skin easily and is a useful moisturiser. A few may be allergic to lanolin, but most allergic reactions come from other ingredients found in cosmetics such as synthetic fragrances and preservatives. A bland, purified lanolin cream is available from most chemists and is a useful ingredient for many skin-soothing recipes.

Magnesia

This alkaline white powder is named after the ancient city of Magnesia in Asia Minor. Often added to stomach upset remedies, it has a drying and tightening effect on the skin. Useful for dabbing neat on to spots and pimples, magnesia can also be found in skin fresheners, anti-perspirants and talcum powders.

Mineral Oil

Made from highly refined petroleum, mineral oil is found in baby oils, baby lotions and commercial cold creams. Unfortunately, when it is heated it gives off a distinctive petrol aroma. A pure, bland product with a lengthy shelf-life, mineral oil crops up in literally thousands of cosmetic and toiletry preparations. It leaves a characteristic film on the skin and does not penetrate the surface. Some dermatologists advise sensitive and acne-prone patients to avoid mineral oil as it can cause an allergic reaction on the skin. Plant oils, such as avocado oil, can be used instead, as these sink more deeply into the skin and contain more nourishing ingredients such as natural vitamins and moisturising essential fatty acids.

Orris Root

This fragrant root or rhizome is an important ingredient in perfume-making as it is used as a fixative for fine fragrances. Orris root comes from the dried rhizome of the *Iris florentina* and is an expensive commodity. This is because it takes four years to grow the rhizomes and two more years to dry them out before they can be used. Ground orris root is useful as a natural talcum powder and a dry hair shampoo. It can also be added to homemade pot-pourri blends as a perfume fixative.

Petroleum Jelly

Also known as petrolatum, this jelly is produced as a by-product of the petroleum industry and is obtained by treating petrol with steam and filtering at high temperatures. Technically, petroleum jelly is a purified mixture of semi-solid hydrocarbons from petroleum. Some may also have an understandable aversion to putting a by-product of petrol on to their skin. Petroleum jelly is extremely thick and works well as a barrier cream, lip salve or a base for homemade ointments.

Pumice

This grey stone consists mainly of silicates and can be found on the beaches of most Greek islands. It has abrasive properties and is used in tooth whiteners, skin scrubs and cleansing grains. Natural pumice stones are often sold to remove the dead, hardened skin on the soles of the feet. These stones are made when the pumice solidifies into small grey lumps thrown out from the many active volcanoes in and around Greece.

Rhassoul Mud

This fine, powdered clay comes from Morocco, where it is mined in the Atlas mountains. It is useful for its de-greasing properties and can be added to hair and body packs to remove excess dirt and sebum. It can also be added to scalp treatments to help severe cases of dandruff and flaking scalps and works by drawing out impurities from the hair follicles. Dried Rhassoul mud is available in small packets from healthfood shops and herbal suppliers, and is a useful substitute for other types of powdered clays such as kaolin or Fuller's earth.

Wheatgerm Oil

Another important beautycare ingredient, wheatgerm oil is our richest natural source of Vitamin E. It comes from the seed or 'germ' of the wheat stalk and is also rich in many vitamins and essential fatty acids that strengthen the skin. Wheatgerm oil is rich and sticky and too concentrated to use on its own or for massage, but a small amount can be added to skin creams and lotions. In addition to enriching a recipe, wheatgerm oil also acts as a natural preservative and its Vitamin E content will prevent the cream from becoming rancid. Wheatgerm oil is also one of the best anti-ageing ingredients as its high Vitamin E content helps neutralise the destructive particles known as free radicals within the skin. These elements are responsible for most of the skin's visible signs of premature ageing, including loss of skin tone and wrinkles. Wheatgerm oil has a distinctive, nutty aroma which you either love or loathe. Either way, a few drops added to skin creams and massage oil blends make one of the most useful of all beauty ingredients.

Zinc Oxide

This thick white paste was the original total sunblock and it can still be used to screen out virtually all of the sun's harmful rays. Zinc oxide has astringent properties, and also dries the skin. It can help healing and is often found in nappy rash creams, anti-perspirants and shaving creams.

These ingredients are from the kitchen cupboard.

Arrowroot

This culinary thickener is used in soups, sauces and gravies but also crops up in talcum powders and hair dyes. Arrowroot comes from the starchy roots of a tropical plant that is common in the West Indies. It was first used by native American Indians to heal wounds inflicted by poisoned arrows. Nowadays, arrowroot is added to moisturisers to make them thicker and to help the active ingredients penetrate the upper levels of the skin.

Beeswax

Commonly found in furniture polish, beeswax also plays an important role in keeping our complexion polished and protected. Beeswax comes from the hexagonal honeycombs in which bees store their honey and flower pollen. Each hexagonal cell is sealed with a fine sheet of beeswax to protect and preserve the honey inside. Beeswax itself is used in many cosmetic preparations, such as moisturising creams, mascara and other kinds of make-up. It has a thick, waxy texture and is good for using on chapped areas of exposed skin, such as the hands and lips. It is available either in small honey-coloured blocks from healthfood shops, or as easy-to-melt granules for cosmetic and candle-making, sold by a herbal supplier.

Brewer's Yeast

This vitamin-enriched food supplement is an excellent source of the important B vitamins, especially thiamin, riboflavin and nicotinic acid. Brewer's yeast is often added to face masks and hair packs for its deeply nourishing properties. It tends to be expensive, if bought in capsule form, but it is much cheaper if you buy packets of dried brewer's yeast from healthfood shops. This is a handy form for beauty recipes and is a useful ingredient for enriching face masks and moisturising creams.

Carrageen Moss

Technically a seaweed, this is also known as Irish moss as it grows mainly around the west coast of Ireland. It has powerful gelling properties and crops up in countless cosmetic preparations, from toothpaste to toilet soap. Carrageen moss contains a type of ingredient known in herbalism as a *mucilage*, meaning that it can be made into a jelly or thick paste. For this reason it is used to thicken many skin creams, gels and face masks. The mucilage in carrageen moss helps relieve skin irritations by forming a protective layer over delicate mucous membranes, and can rapidly relieve inflammation. Medical herbalists may also use carrageen moss internally to treat persistent coughs or peptic (stomach) ulcers. Dehydrated carrageen moss is available from supermarkets and healthfood shops.

Cornflour

Also known as cornstarch, this is made from finely ground maize or sweetcorn kernels and often crops up in talcum powder and fine face powder. Highly absorbent, it is useful as a homemade anti-perspirant and can be used on its own or blended with rice flour or arrowroot.

Corn Oil

This vegetable oil is extracted from ripened corn kernels, and is also known as maize oil. Unrefined corn oil, from healthfood shops, contains high levels of Vitamin E, which make it a useful body moisturiser. Corn oil is thicker than most other vegetable oils and should be used sparingly in beauty recipes to prevent stickiness.

Gelatine

This jelling agent is obtained by boiling the skin, tendons, ligaments and bones of animal carcasses with water. Gelatine attracts moisture and is able to absorb between five to ten times its own weight in water. It is used in protein shampoos because it gives the hair more 'body', and is also the main ingredient in peel-off face masks and some fingernail strengtheners. Carageen moss may be used as an alternative, vegetable-based gelling agent.

Grapeseed Oil

Grapeseed oil is a light, colourless oil that is extracted from grape pips. Because it is highly refined, grapeseed oil has a fine texture and is odourless, making it one of the best plant oils for massage. Many aromatherapists use grapeseed oil to blend with essential oils before massage treatments. Grapeseed oil is also a useful ingredient of body lotions and lightweight skin creams.

Groundnut Oil

Also known as peanut oil, this oil comes from peanut kernels. The peanut is not actually a nut, but the seed pod of a legume that grows beneath the ground. Common in Africa, India and China, peanuts are a rich source of protein and produce a nutritious oil that is a valuable source of Vitamin E. Unrefined groundnut oil, from healthfood shops, is the best type to use in beauty recipes as this retains most of its natural nutrients.

Hazelnut Oil

One of the newest plant oils to appear on the supermarket shelves, hazelnut oil is made from pressed hazelnut kernels. The best quality oil comes from France, where much of it is still produced in old-fashioned, family-run oil mills. Hazelnut oil has good penetrating powers and is one of the best oils to use on the skin. Pharmacist Claudine Luu, who runs courses on natural medicine at Montpelier University in France, recommends using hazelnut oil as a base for essential oil massage. She says it is especially good for treating conditions such as abscesses, acne and sore throats, where the essential oils are required to quickly penetrate the surface of the skin.

Honey

Made by bees from the sweet nectar in plants and flowers, honey itself is a mixture of ninety-eight per cent sugars, with two per cent enzymes, vitamins and minerals. It has mildly antiseptic properties, meaning that bacterium cannot survive in it. There are several different types of honey, and its colour is largely affected by the kinds of blossom that the bees visit to produce it. The best-quality honey is also slightly cloudy, which means that it retains the vitamin-enriched pollen that contributes to its nutrient content. The darker-coloured honeys have higher levels of minerals and are probably better to use in skincare recipes. Honey is a useful soothing ingredient in moisturisers, hand creams and body lotions, but it is best avoided if you are allergic to pollen or grasses.

Kelp

Also known as bladderwrack, kelp is often used as a generic name for all kinds of seaweed and can be found in most good healthfood shops. Dehydrated kelp can be bought in packets to use as a vegetable, or in powder form, either loose or in capsules. It should not be used fresh from the beach unless you are sure that the waters from which it came are unpolluted. Rich in vitamins and marine minerals, kelp is a useful ingredient in face masks and treatments for several skin problems, including psoriasis. As with carrageen moss, another type of seaweed, kelp is rich in mucilage or gelling agents. It is widely used by medical herbalists to treat sluggishness and joint inflammations such as arthritis. It is also used for thyroid conditions because of its high iodine content and is known as the slimmer's friend, as it stimulates thyroid activity which in turn peps up a sluggish metabolism.

Lecithin

Lecithin is an essential fatty acid found in egg yolks, soya beans, avocados and unrefined cooking oils. In humans, lecithin is found in the membranes of all our cells and it is a vital component of skin tissue, helping to keep the complexion strong and healthy. One of the easiest ways to use lecithin in cosmetic recipes is in the form of egg yolks, which contain around ten per cent pure lecithin. It can also be bought in powdery granules or in capsules from a chemist or healthfood shop. Lecithin is one of the skin's own Natural Moisturising Factors (NMFs) which are found in the lower levels of the skin. Other NMFs include urea compounds, lactic acid and glycolic acid. Lecithin acts as an emulsifier, holding a liquid in a suspension to prevent it separating. This is why egg yolks are used in making mayonnaise – to bind together the oil and vinegar. Lecithin is a useful skincare ingredient and is often added to moisturisers, as it helps lock moisture into the skin.

Linseeds

Also known as flaxseeds, these come from the flax plant, which used to be a common sight in Britain during Anglo-Saxon times when it was grown to produce flax linen. The seeds themselves are small, brown and shiny, and have an oily taste, due to their extremely high natural oil content. Linseeds are also rich in mucilage and waxes and can be used to make natural gels and thick pastes for beauty recipes. Linseeds can also be used internally as a safe, effective remedy for constipation, and make good internal cleansers (simply swallow a handful followed by a large glass of water to encourage the seeds to swell up and pass quickly through the digestive tract). Medical herbalists also use linseeds internally to relieve rasping coughs or to draw out boils and other types of severe skin inflammations. Linseeds may also be used in poultices to heal burns, scalds and boils.

Maple Syrup

Natural maple syrup comes from the sap of the Canadian maple tree or *Acer saccarum*. It is a natural source of sugars that are similar to those needed by the skin to maintain its moisture content. Pure maple syrup (not to be confused with the more common synthetic version) has moisturising and slightly antiseptic properties, and can be used in recipes instead of honey.

Oatmeal

Oats are a good source of protein, vitamins and, perhaps surprisingly, polyunsaturated fats. They are also extremely soothing on the skin and are perfect ingredients for treating overly dry, irritated or sensitive skin conditions. There are several different types of oatmeal that may be used success-fully in skincare recipes and all are available from supermarkets or healthfood shops. Porridge oat flakes are useful for adding to a warm bath to soften the water and help restore moisture to the skin. Coarsely ground and medium ground oatmeal make good exfoliating skin scrubs, while fine ground oatmeal is better for treatments on areas of more delicate skin, such as the face and neck.

Olive Oil

Not only is olive oil the best type of oil for cooking, it is also an essential ingredient of many beauty recipes. One reason is that, unlike other vegetable oils, olive oil remains stable when heated to high temperatures and also resists rancidity. Olive oil has been used in skincare for thousands of years (the father of medicine, Hippocrates, said that it should be rubbed on to sunburn to help heal inflamed skin). There are two main types of olive oil that you can buy from the super-market. Extra virgin oil is the best quality, as it contains the first pressing of the olives and has not been chemically re-fined. In fact, this is one of the few truly natural ingredients still found on the supermarket shelves. Extra virgin olive oil also contains the most Vitamin E and lecithin. Its dis-advantage is that it also has a distinctive, olivey smell which can be off-putting. Pure olive oil, sold as a liquid laxative, is often a better choice for beauty recipes, as it is a more refined version with a finer texture and little fragrance. Highly purified olive oil is also available in small bottles from the chemist, and this may be used if you want to avoid all traces of odour.

Propolis

This is another by-product of the industrious honey bees. Propolis is the brown, gum-like substance that bees make by collecting sap from tree buds and mix with their own secretions to paint the inside of their hives and mummify the remains of any intruders. Propolis is highly antiseptic and has remarkable anti-bacterial properties which repel bacterial and fungal infections on the skin. It is also reputed to strengthen the human immune system by encouraging the thymus gland to produce extra white blood cells. Propolis has mild painkilling properties and can be found in healthfood shops in the form of a spray for a sore-throat, or soothing lozenges.

Rice Flour

A fine, creamy-coloured flour made from ground rices, this has an unusually silky texture. Highly absorbent and drying on the skin, rice flour is often used in face and body powders and is available from good healthfood shops. Pure rice flour is a useful substitute for talcum powder and can be scented with the addition of a few drops of aromatic essential oils.

Royal Jelly

Royal jelly is made by the worker bees as food to fatten up the Queen Bee and sustain her supply of larvae. As worker bees live for about six weeks and the Queen can live for up to six years (despite laying around 2000 eggs a day), royal jelly is obviously powerful stuff. Little is known about the exact attributes of this remarkable substance. Technically, royal jelly contains traces of all the B Vitamins, Vitamin C, twenty-two amino acids, numerous minerals, enzymes and trace elements, plus a mysterious four per cent which has defied analysis. Royal jelly is often added to skincare ranges and is said to have miraculous anti-ageing properties, although the tiny amounts added to commercial skincare products means it would have minimal effect. While it is unlikely that royal jelly will turn back the clock, it may help to reduce dryness and sensitivity in some skintypes. It can be bought in capsule form and the contents of these is a useful ingredient for adding to face masks and enriching skin creams.

Sesame Oil

One of the earliest plant oils to be used in health and beauty remedies, sesame oil can be traced back to Roman times. The oil comes from the plant's tiny seeds, which themselves are a good source of iron, calcium and protein. Sesame oil is soothing on the skin and has little or no smell, making it a good choice for many beauty recipes.

Sunflower Oil

This popular vegetable oil comes from the seeds in the head of the sunflower plant, which is grown throughout America and Europe for its valuable oil. An attractive, fast-growing plant, sunflowers can also be grown in the garden. Once the seeds have ripened and turned black they can be collected and eaten as a nutritious snack. The vivid yellow flower petals may also be dried and used to make a natural blonde hair dye. Sunflower oil is best bought in an unrefined state from a healthfood shop, as this contains higher levels of nutrients, including Vitamin E and calcium. It is a useful and inexpensive basic oil for massage blends and body lotions.

Walnut Oil

An expensive oil that contains high levels of Vitamin E and other useful skin nutrients, walnut oil is sometimes known by its French name *huile de noix*. Walnut oil can be found in healthfood shops or on some supermarket shelves. It is made from warm-pressing walnut kernels, which are naturally rich in this golden oil. Walnut oil can be used in skincare blends and is a useful alternative to almond or hazelnut oil.

Vanilla Pods

These long dark beans are a member of the orchid family and can be found on the shelves of delicatessens and healthfood shops. Vanilla pods have been valued for their exotic fragrance for centuries and were first used by the Aztecs to fragrance body creams and perfumes. The pods are very expensive but can be used again and again to give a warm, subtle aroma to skincare recipes. Whenever you use a pod, rinse it well, dry thoroughly and return to an airtight container. Alternatively, a few drops of natural vanilla essence will give a similar velvety scent to products like body lotions and hand creams.

Vinegar

Each country develops its own type of vinegar according to the local alcoholic drinks – wine vinegars in France, rice vinegars in Japan and malt vinegar based on beer in Britain. Although it is our home-brew, malt vinegar should not be used on the skin as it is far too harsh, and overpoweringly pungent. The best form of vinegar for skincare products, such as skin tonics, is natural cider vinegar which has a relatively low acidity. Cider vinegar contains around five per cent malic acid, which is similar to the hydrochloric acid produced by the stomach and used to digest food. Cider vinegar is useful for restoring the correct acid pH balance to skin fresheners and for adding to the final rinsing water after shampooing as it gives gleaming highlights to the hair.

3

The Botanicals

In addition to the basic range of raw materials needed to make preparations to cleanse and protect our skin and hair, there is also a range of natural plant extracts that can be added to give products specific benefits. For example, a skin tonic may be created to suit a dry, sensitive skin by adding chamomile flowers, or a product may be made suitable for an oily, combination skin by including nettles and yarrow.

The Romans were largely responsible for bringing many Mediterranean plants and herbs to Britain and for their subsequent wide-scale cultivation. They encouraged the use of plants and herbs in health and beauty preparations, as well as in perfumes and as salad or cooking ingredients. After the Roman Empire collapsed, herbs and herbal medicines fell out of favour, encouraged by the rise in Christianity which considered faith, penitence and prayer to be the only answers to illness. Herbs then became associated with witchcraft and many of the original herbalists had a difficult time in re-establishing their art.

However, many herbs and plants remain potent natural healers and have a wide range of uses in beauty preparations. For example, a variety of bullwort has been used for centuries for skin and kidney complaints, and it is now used in hospitals, together with ultra-violet light therapy, to treat severe skin conditions such as psoriasis and vitiligo. Even on a day-to-day level most modern skincare products still rely on herbal extracts that have been tried and tested over literally thousands of years.

The simplest way to ensure a steady supply of fresh herbs and plants, such as roses and geraniums, is to grow your own, either in the garden, in a window box or along a sunny window sill. Many extracts come from plants normally classed as weeds, such as stinging nettles, and these are remarkably easy to grow. In fact, without careful control, they will quickly take over the flowerbeds. Many flowers also have unusual properties that are especially useful in skincare. For example, marigolds give us a soothing calendula extract and geranium leaves contain one of the best natural perfumes.

When picking herbs and wild plants, avoid those that have been growing along a roadside or close to any source of industrial pollution. Plants are highly sensitive to pollutants in the atmosphere and quickly absorb them into their petals and leaves. If growing or gathering your own supplies sounds too much like hard work, dried herbs and flower heads are readily available from herbal suppliers (there is a comprehensive list of these, including mail-order details, at the back of this book). Fresh herbs are also increasingly available from supermarkets and grocers, but do not be tempted to use flowers from the florist as these blooms are often sprayed with powerful herbicides which will harm the skin. The most useful plants for cosmetic and beauty preparations are listed alphabetically below.

Arnica *Arnica montana*

Also known as leopard's bane, this vivid yellow alpine flower has many well-documented medicinal uses. The arnica flower looks like a spindly yellow daisy, but it is the plant's roots that are of most use to us. From the root we can extract tincture of arnica, a powerful compound containing the bitter yellow substance called arnicin. Unlike its flowers, the root also contains tannins as well as several minerals. Tincture of arnica is available from most chemists and is extremely useful for applying to bruises (every first-aid kit should contain a bottle). It works by stimulating the circulation, and arnica cream is one of the most effective remedies for preventing a bruise from turning blue. Tincture of arnica is toxic, so it is for external use only and must not be swallowed. However, an extremely diluted form of arnica in tablet form is available from homoeopathic suppliers, and this is an excellent remedy for shock, or any emotional or physical injury. A safe, effective treatment, arnica tablets are especially recommended for children's bruises, childbirth and minor accidents. Further details of homoeopathic suppliers and practitioners can be found at the back of this book.

Chamomile (German) *Matricaria chamomilla*

This herb takes its name from the Greek *kamai* (ground) and *melon* (apple), because of the sweet apple-like fragrance it releases when trodden on. Traditionally used to make scented lawns, chamomile is a low-growing, ground-covering herb with many practical uses. There are many varieties, including *Anthemis nobilis*, used for the lawns at Buckingham Palace, but aromatherapists prefer *Matricaria chamomilla*, or German chamomile, which produces a highly prized blue oil. The secret to this plant's success are substances called *azulenes* which have skin-soothing and anti-inflammatory properties. For this reason a synthetic form of azulene is often found in commercial skincare products such as eye gels.

Natural German chamomile also contains another extract called alpha-bisabolol, which is used in many skincare preparations for its uniquely soothing action on the skin. Studies at the University of Bonn in Germany have shown alpha-bisabolol to have both painkilling and anti-inflammatory properties. Trials have illustrated that it helps repair sun-damaged and chemically injured skin tissues, and that there is a proven basis for using chamomile extract to help wound healing.

The medicinal properties of natural chamomile are concentrated in the yellow centre of its flowers, and this is the part that is dried and turned into a sedative herb tea. Other parts of the plant, such as the whole flower heads and the leaves, are useful as a tonic and can be added to a bath to relieve tired, aching muscles.

Chamomile flowers are also useful as a gentle hair dye and bring a glossy sheen to naturally blonde hair. Chamomile tea-bags are a useful and convenient way of making herbal infusions and also make a soothing drink that helps the digestion. Medical herbalists often use chamomile internally to treat tension headaches, insomnia and nervous digestive disorders. The herb is also used frequently in children's remedies as it can help to calm and relieve many infant conditions including colic, teething and hyperactivity. Pure chamomile concentrate is available in liquid form from healthfood shops for adding to skincare recipes or using in healing compresses.

Chrysanthemum *Chrysanthemum morifolium*

This popular garden flower is cultivated in China purely for its medicinal properties. Herbalism has been popular in the Far East for at least the last 5000 years and relies on Oriental herbs and plants for its medicines. The principle of this form of herbalism is prevention rather than cure by achieving an internal *yin-yang* balance (where the body is in a state of perfect harmony with no sign of stress or strain).

The idea of yin and yang was developed around 100 BC by Dong Zhongshu. He documented the balance of opposing principles (yin-yang) as applied to the body. 'Cold' herbs and foods (yin) were identified to correct 'hot' conditions or diseases, and vice versa. The principles of balancing foods in this way is still practised by most of China's one billion inhabitants.

Chrysanthemum petals contain useful essential oils which have sedative and soothing properties. In Chinese medicine they are prescribed for headaches, influenza, hypertension and atherosclerosis (hardening of the arteries). An infusion is used as an eye bath for disorders such as conjunctivitis and it is used in compresses to treat abscesses. An infusion can be made using fresh flower heads or chrysanthemum tea bags (from healthfood shops) and makes an astringent skin tonic.

Chrysanthemum tea combines many of the soothing benefits of drinking chamomile tea, but tastes better because it does not contain the glycoside called anthemic acid that gives chamomile its slightly bitter taste.

Comfrey *Symphytum officinale*

A tall herb that is best suited to growing outdoors in the back of a flower bed or in the vegetable patch, comfrey is the friend of the organic gardener. Russian comfrey or the *S. peri-grinum* variety is often grown specifically to be turned into a nutrient-rich compost for fertilising the soil. Comfrey contains many vitamins, minerals and trace elements that are ideal for replenishing nutrients in the earth. It also contains *allantoin*, which is extracted from its roots and used as an effective skin soother and healer. For this reason, allantoin extracts are often added to ointments to help eczema and psoriasis. Comfrey is also used to heal wounds, stomach ulcers and bone fractures as it contains agents that bind together tissues while also stimulating new growth. However, although comfrey has many uses on the surface of the skin it should be taken internally with *great* care. Comfrey contains powerful alkaloids that affect the liver and there have been reports of poisoning from drinking large amounts of comfrey tea. Alkaloids are organic compounds that contain nitrogen and include atropine, a poison found in deadly nightshade: caffeine and theobromide, found in coffee; morphine found in the opium poppy; and solanine found in poisonous green potatoes.

Many herbs and plant extracts can have a powerful effect within the body and should only be taken internally in large doses when under the guidance of a qualified medical herbalist. For our purposes in beauty remedies it is best to confine comfrey to external applications only.

Cornflower *Centaurea cyanus*

A plant that likes to grow in or near cornfields, hence its name, the cornflower is easily recognised by its vivid blue flowers. The petals provide a deep blue dye that is used to make ink and water-colour paints. Cornflower extract also comes from its blue petals and has mildly antibiotic properties, which are used to soothe the skin. An infusion of flower heads in distilled water makes a mildly astringent skin tonic. Cornflower lotions are also especially soothing around the eye area and the extract is often added to expensive eye creams.

Cowslip *Primula veris*

A small wild flower with a tall stem topped with a dozen or so vivid yellow blooms, the cowslip plant has a sweet smell, due to the anethol content in its stems and roots. Its name comes from the Anglo Saxon *cusloppe*, meaning cow's slobber. Cowslip has been used in medical herbalism for centuries for its stimulating expectorant, anti-spasmodic and sedative properties. It is still possible to buy herbal cough mixtures containing cowslip extracts and these are especially useful to treat children with bronchitis or whooping cough.

Cowslips are also used to treat nervous excitement and to help insomnia. According to the English herbalist Culpeper, writing in 1653, an infusion of cowslip petals will 'take away spots and wrinkles of the skin, sun-burning and freckles, and doth add beauty exceedingly'. Culpeper also used a mixture of cowslip leaves and hog's grease for soothing burns and wounds.

Slightly more appealing is a mixture used in skincare remedies for centuries, made from petals that have been infused in almond or olive oil. When analysed, the flowers have been found to be mildly diuretic, anti-inflammatory and anti-spasmodic. They are also useful in skincare for sensitive skins, as they can reduce the amount of histamine released by the body and so cut down on allergic reactions.

Dandelion *Taraxacum officinale*

This plant gets its name from the French words for lion's tooth *dent de lion*. It was given this nickname by ancient herbalists who considered it to be as powerful as the teeth of the lion when it comes to tackling disorders of the human body. Dandelion leaves are highly nutritious and one of our richest sources of iron and potassium, together with numerous other vitamins and minerals. Instead of spraying the dandelions in your lawn with weedkiller, a better option would be to pick the leaves when they are young and tender and add them to a salad. Dandelion leaves can also be covered by a bucket while they are still growing, to blanch them and reduce their bitterness. The leaves may also be collected, dried and made into a tea, which has mild diuretic properties.

Dandelion root is also highly prized by medical herbalists as a digestive, a liver tonic and a natural laxative. It is also used to treat skin problems such as eczema and inflammation, and conditions including jaundice. In addition, the white sap from the plant's stalks is reputed to be an effective long-term remedy for removing warts.

Eyebright *Euphrasia officinalis*

A small pretty plant with dainty dark green leaves and bluish white flowers, eyebright is an alpine herb, that rarely grows taller than five ins (18 cms). Eyebright always grows on grass, which it relies on for providing part of its food supply. It is so-called due to its effectiveness at clearing the eyes and preventing soreness.

The homoeopathic 'Tincture of Euphrasia' is excellent for treating eye disorders such as conjunctivitis, or swollen, sticky eyes associated with hay fever and allergies. To use, dilute one drop in a sterile eye-bath with distilled or boiled, cooled water. Use to bathe the eyes three times a day, using a different eye-bath for each eye to prevent cross-infection. As homemade infusions of eyebright may not be sufficiently sterile to use directly in the eyes, it is best to use 'Tincture of Euphrasia' or a professional liquid decoction of the herb. Eyebright may also be used in compresses to relieve tired, red eyes and is often added to commercial eye drops and eye gels for this reason.

Fennel *Foeniculum vulgare*

Fennel was named after the Latin word for hay, as it was thought to have the same scent as freshly mown hay. When Pliny the Elder wrote on the merits of herbs, he detailed twenty-two different curative effects of fennel. He had observed a snake rubbing its eyes on the plant and came to the conclusion that fennel was therefore good for the eyes. Two thousand years later, fennel is still associated with the eyes and an infusion made from the seeds is useful for making a compress to treat tired and sore eyes. Fennel is also reputed to be the 'herb of immortality' and is associated with ageing well and longevity.

The main component of fennel oil is anethol, which is used to perfume toiletries such as shampoo and soap (see *Essential Oils*, page 63).

Fennel tea also contains a small amount of the natural plant oils and is useful for expelling wind from the system, for cases of persistent hiccups and to pep up a weak digestive system. Fennel is commonly used to make gripe water, a childhood remedy for colic, and can help cases of flatulence and other intestinal disturbances. The essential oils contained in fennel have constituents similar to adrenalin, which may be why it has a tonic effect on the digestion and can stimulate the appetite. Fennel is traditionally an anti-nauseant, and is often used to relieve morning sickness in pregnancy and motion sickness. It is also useful for relieving inflammations of mucous membranes such as the eyes and mouth, and is a time-honoured remedy for increasing milk production when breastfeeding.

Geranium *Pelargonium capitatum*

This well-known flowering plant is unusual because its scent is found mainly in the leaves and not its attractive red and pink flowers. Depending upon the variety, geranium leaves may smell of peppermint, rose, orange, spices or even pineapple. All types are good to grow in the garden or in pots as they provide an attractive display of colour during the summer months and need almost no looking after. *Pelargonium capitatum* is the variety most widely used in cosmetics as its leaves contain a rose scent, due to an alcohol called geraniol, which is also found in roses.

Frequently used as a cheaper alternative to pure rose oil which has become prohibitively expensive (see also *Essential Oils*, page 64), this extract is gentle on the skin and can be used in moisturisers and skin lotions for dry and sensitive complexions. The roots of wild geraniums (*Geranium maculatum*) are also used internally by medical herbalists for their astringent properties to treat diarrhoea and bowel diseases.

Lavender *Lavendula officinalis*

The word lavender was coined in the Middle Ages and comes from the Latin verb *lavare*, meaning to wash or clean. Lavender has been a popular herb in Britain for centuries and the use of this purple-flowered spiky plant dates back to the late sixteenth century. Lavender gets its distinctive smell from the small green pods that sit on either side of the small purple flowers. These pods contain the plant's essential oil, which has many medicinal properties. Medical herbalists may use lavender to treat irritability, stress and depression, and the oil can be used neat on the skin to help heal burns and wounds (see *Essential Oils*, page 65).

Lavender should be gathered in July or August, just before the flowers have fully opened, and spread out to dry in a warm place away from direct sunlight, which fades the flowers. When dry, the aromatic flower heads easily rub off between the fingers and thumb. These can be kept in a tightly sealed jar and used to make infusions or to fragrance pot-pourri.

Lemon Balm *Melissa officinalis*

This easy-to-grow herb looks like mint but has highly perfumed leaves which give off a lemon scent when crushed between the fingers. Lemon balm thrives in most soils and will grow up to three ft (90 cm) high and, unlike common mint, its roots do not spread very far. The plant takes its botanical name from the Greek *melissa*, which means honey. This is because its tiny white flowers are an attractive source of nectar for the honey bee. Used by medical herbalists as a relaxant, lemon balm tea can be a useful drink when feeling anxious or tense. Melissa oil comes from the plant's leaves and was an important ingredient in Carmelite water, one of the first commercial perfumes made by Carmelite monks in medieval Europe (see *Essential Oils*, page 67).

Marigold *Calendula officinalis*

Also known as pot marigold, this plant derives its botanical name from its flowers, which often bloom on the first day of the month, a time formerly known as the *calends*. In Anglo Saxon days, marigolds were woven into garlands for feasts and weddings, as their golden colour symbolised strength and healing. The petals were also used to treat jaundice, headaches and sore, red eyes. The flower heads have distinctive orange petals which can be collected and used as a natural hair dye. The petals may also be scattered on to salads as an attractive garnish, and have a slightly bitter flavour.

One of the most useful skincare extracts is calendula oil, which is extracted from the petals by steeping them for a fortnight in pure vegetable oil, such as almond or olive oil. This contains natural steroid substances called *sterols* and is especially good for treating skin conditions like eczema, or cases where the skin has been damaged by steroid abuse.

A half and half mixture of calendula oil and St John's wort oil is an especially effective remedy for repairing scarred or damaged skin. This type of flower petal maceration also provides a rich source of beta carotene, a vitamin vitally important for healthy skin tissues. It is especially useful to boost the vitamin content of homemade moisturisers.

The juice from marigold petals can also be squeezed from the flower heads and used neat on spots and insect bites. Herbalists only use the petals of the marigold flower and favour the *officinalis* variety, which is available dried from herbal suppliers (this should not be confused with the many tpes of cultivated marigolds that are grown for the garden). Marigold tincture is also available and this can be mixed with equal parts of witch hazel to make a tonic for irritated, sensitive skins.

Mint *Mentha piperita*

Discovered by British botanist John Rea in 1700, this herb is named for its peppery smell. There are many varieties of mint including peppermint, spearmint and eau de cologne mint. The best to grow for beauty recipes is peppermint or *Mentha piperita*. This variety has one of the strongest aromas and also works well in recipes for cooking. When planting mint in the garden it is advisable to place it in a bucket first before sinking it into the soil, otherwise its roots quickly spread and the plant takes over the entire garden.

Peppermint has many health and beauty benefits, and it crops up in countless preparations. Peppermint oil contains many substances including turpentine and menthol, which gives it a camphor-like smell. Cold on the skin, menthol is often included in refreshing skin tonics and invigorating shower foams. Traditionally used in toothpastes to refresh the mouth and teeth, menthol also numbs the gums and can relieve toothache.

Peppermint has a good influence on the metabolism and peppermint tea is often drunk to improve the flow of bile to the liver, resulting in the correct digestion of fats. Being an astringent herb, peppermint tea is also useful in treating nausea and digestive upsets, and medical herbalists may use peppermint internally to relieve irritable bowel syndrome and dyspepsia. Peppermint leaves have a bitter taste which means they contain elements that stimulate important digestive enzymes within the body. Recent research shows that oil of peppermint (which is contained to some degree in peppermint tea) can be used to treat irritable bowel syndrome and it is currently on trial in some hospitals (see also *Essential Oils*, page 68).

Plantain *Plantago major*

A common sight in British hedgerows, plantain is a small weed that can be recognised by its oval ribbed leaves and short seed stalks that resemble rat's tails. Plaintain often grows alongside stinging nettles and is the natural antidote to their sting. The herbalist Nicholas Culpeper had many uses for plantain and said that the plant's juice cleared up intestinal disorders and helped women with abormally heavy periods. He used the roots of the plant to cure toothache and its seeds for treating consumption. The juice was also recommended for disorders as diverse as piles and lunacy!

These days we are more likely to confine our use of plantain to rubbing the longer leaves or the juice from the stalks on to nettle rash to take away the itch and swelling. However, plantain juice is also an all-round skin soother and an infusion can be made by boiling clean leaves in milk to use on sunburn or chapped skin. It is a good source of the minerals zinc and silica, both of which are needed to maintain skin strength and suppleness. Medical herbalists may use extracts made from dried plantain leaves to treat cases of skin irritation and inflammation, such as allergic skin rashes and haemorrhoids (piles). These extracts have been shown to have anti-microbial effects and Chinese medicine also uses plantain to treat urinary disorders and kidney problems.

Primrose *Primula vulgaris*

Primrose is another wild plant native to Britain that has excellent skincare properties. The primrose plant produces its flowers in early spring and so takes its name from the Latin *primus*, meaning first. The juice from the primrose leaves was used by herbalists for many years as an astringent skin tonic, and Culpeper commented that primrose ointment made from the leaves was an excellent salve for sore skins. In his

Complete Herbal, written in 1653, he urges, 'do not see your poor neighbour go with wounded limbs when a halfpenny cost (for primrose salve) will heal them'. In herbalism, the roots and leaves of the primrose are the only parts that are used. These contain anti-inflammatory and anti-spasmodic extracts which used to be common cures for rheumatism, gout, insomnia and as a poultice to heal burns and wounds.

Rose *Rosa Damascena*

Called the Queen of Flowers, it is hard to beat the rose for its perfume and sheer beauty. Of the many varieties of roses grown in Britain it is the *Rosa damascena* that gives us some of the most wonderful scent. Originally from the Middle East, legend has it that this variety was born from a single drop of sweat falling from Mohammed's brow. It also gave its name to the town of Damascus in Syria, which was famed for damask silk woven in colours to match the flowers. One of the earliest records of the damask rose was by Greek historian Herodotus, who wrote that the flower had some sixty petals and a scent to surpass all others. First used in perfumery, pure rose oil is frighteningly expensive as it takes around 250lbs (110kg) of petals to produce a single ounce of concentrated essential oil. Still cultivated in a few areas such as Grasse in southern France, the rose petals must be picked by hand early in the morning before the sun rises high in the sky and evaporates the oil.

In addition to rose oil, rosewater is also a by-product of the distillation process that produces the essential oil (see page 69). This is a more common ingredient in skincare and a version can be made at home by steeping clean rose petals in water. Note that the rosewater commonly available from chemists is more frequently made with synthetic fragrance extracts, not roses. Genuine rosewater is available from herbal and aromatherapy suppliers and contains up to twenty per cent pure essential oils that are soluble in water and therefore left behind after the distillation process.

Rosemary *Rosmarinus officinalis*

Named from the Latin *ros-marinus* which means dew of the sea, rosemary is an attractive evergreen herb with aromatic, needle-shaped leaves. It is popular in cooking, as its strong flavour complements fatty foods such as lamb, or oily fish such as mackerel. Rosemary is rich in fragrant oils that the plant stores in cells, just beneath the leaf surface, visible only with a magnifier. These oils are released in the sunshine or a warm breeze or when the plant is handled (see *Essential Oils*, page 70). A simple rosemary oil maceration can be made by soaking a handful of clean, flowering stalks in a good quality almond or olive oil. Cover tightly and leave for at least a week before filtering the fragrant infusion. Use for rubbing into tired feet, or for adding to a refreshing bath.

Rosemary has invigorating properties and has been used for centuries in beauty preparations, especially hair and scalp remedies. Naturally antiseptic, a rosemary hair rinse can be used to help dandruff and flakiness after the final shampoo.

In *Banck's Herbal*, written in 1525, women are advised to 'smell it oft as it shall keep thee youngly'. Culpeper also recommended rosemary 'to take away spots, marks and scars in the skin'. More recently, rosemary has been found to contain a substance called *diosmin* which helps strengthen fragile capillaries and may even improve disfiguring skin conditions such as broken thread veins. Rosemary tea is also recommended by modern herbalists to help ease migraine and headaches. Herbal extracts containing rosemary may also be prescribed to treat liver problems and nervous disorders.

Sage *Salvia officinalis*

Sage is a small shrubby herb with pale green leaves covered in downy hairs, which give them a greyish tinge. According to an Anglo Saxon manuscript, 'Why should man die when he can have sage?' and from this saying comes its botanical Latin name *salvia* meaning salvation. Sage has many unusual medicinal properties and is a powerful antiseptic (Chinese herbalists even use sage to boost brain power). Modern studies have shown that sage is a natural antibiotic and that it contains hormonal components similar to a vegetable form of oestrogen. For this reason a medical herbalist may use it when treating menstrual disorders, infertility or problems associated with the menopause.

Sage tea is an excellent gargle for sore throats and is made by using one tablespoonful of leaves to each cup, infusing with boiling water for five minutes before straining and gargling (do not swallow). Sage oil is also useful in a massage mixture rubbed into the neck to treat tonsillitis (see *Essential Oils*, page 70). Sage infusions made from the flowering tops of the plant are traditionally used to bring out the lustre of dark hair and can be added to the final rinse water after shampooing.

St John's Wort *Hypericum perforatum*

Named after St John the Baptist, as it usually flowers on his feast day of 24 June, this herb has attractive bright yellow flowers with a cluster of fine stamens. Its small green leaves are dotted with oil glands containing caproic acid which gives off a pungent smell that has been unkindly likened to wet goat's fur. When the leaves are held up to the light they are seen to be full of tiny holes, which is why the French call this herb *Mille-pertuis*, or a thousand perforations. Historically, St John's wort is one of our most useful herbs for health and beauty as it has more medicinal properties than almost any other plant.

When prescribed for internal use by a medical herbalist, St John's wort can treat a range of emotional problems, including anxiety, depression and long-term stress. Externally, the herb has astringent, antiseptic properties and is a mild painkiller. As the plant's flowers also contain oil glands, its petals may be macerated or infused in pure vegetable oil to produce an attractive pink oil. This valuable natural healer can be used on the skin to hasten wound healing and to reduce scarring from burns. It is an excellent addition to any first aid box and is useful in skincare remedies designed for sensitive complexions.

Stinging Nettle *Urtica dioica*

Usually considered to be an unwelcome weed, the stinging nettle has many uses in herbalism. The entire stem and leaves of the plant are covered with tiny stiff hairs which contain formic acid. This is released on to the skin as soon as the plant is touched and causes an allergic reaction. Despite the hazards of their cultivation, stinging nettles can be cooked and eaten just like any other herb. They are best harvested in the spring when the shoots are young and tender. These can be lightly boiled and served like spinach or spring greens (one of Prince Charles's favourite dishes is said to be nettle soup). Rich in Vitamin C and iron, nettles are one of the best sources of chlorophyll, the plant pigment which is similar in structure to the haemoglobin in our red blood cells.

Stinging nettles also have diuretic properties and capsules are often prescribed by medical herbalists for a variety of disorders including anaemia, water retention and gout. They may also use nettles to treat skin problems, such as childhood and allergic eczema, as well as cases of poor circulation. Stinging nettles themselves contain the trace minerals silica and potassium which strengthen the skin, and are used for many skin conditions.

An infusion of the flowering nettle tops sweetened with honey or maple syrup is a useful tonic and internal cleanser as it contains many minerals. It also has substances reputed to cleanse the liver, making it better able to metabolise fats and therefore help purify the complexion from within. Added to skin fresheners, nettles can be used to make a beneficial facial wash with mildly astringent properties. Nettle infusions are also useful as a hair tonic as they add sheen to all hair types and are widely reputed to prevent hair loss.

Sweet Marjoram *Origanum marjorana*

A common culinary herb with tiny white or pink flowers, sweet marjoram is also traditionally used in haircare treatments such as shampoos and scalp lotions. Sweet marjoram has an attractive herby smell that is often used in perfumery, especially for men's aftershave. The oil is extracted from the plant's leaves and young shoots and has antiseptic and antiviral properties (see *Essential Oils*, page 71).

Thyme *Thymus vulgaris*

Thyme is a hardy herb that survives in poor soils and dry climates. Thyme leaves contain a strong antiseptic substance called *thymol*, which is useful in several health and beauty remedies. Thyme oil is used in soaps and added to some skincare preparations for its anti-bacterial properties. The oil is also useful for treating sore throats and a few drops may be mixed with almond oil and rubbed on to the neck to treat tonsillitis. An infusion of thyme leaves also makes a good anti-dandruff scalp tonic (see *Essential Oils*, page 72). Medical herbalists may use thyme to treat a variety of disorders, including respiratory problems, as it acts as a decongestant and expectorant. It has also been used to treat menstrual disorders and mouth infections. Although the chief constituent of thyme oil is thymol it also contains *borneol* and *linalol*, which give it a pleasanter smell. Not all creatures find the scent attractive, though, and sachets of dried thyme mixed with lavender and placed amongst clothes are a useful way of deterring insects and fabric-eating moths.

Violet *Viola odorata*

This wonderful little wild flower prefers to grow in cool, damp conditions and can often be found in woodlands, where it enjoys the moist, leafy soil. The heart-shaped leaves of the violet plant are dark green and it has tiny dark purple flowers, often hidden by the larger foliage. The violet is well known for its sweet, heady fragrance, which sadly fades as soon as the flowers are picked. This is due to its chemical composition which contains the volatile substance *ionine*, from which the name violet is derived. Violet herbal extracts have anti-inflammatory properties and are useful as a skin soother. A diluted version can also be used as a mouthwash for throat and mouth infections. Medical herbalists may use extracts from the flowers and leaves internally, as a powerful expectorant to treat respiratory and lung disorders.

Witch Hazel *Hamamelis virginiana*

A shrubby plant originating from the east coast of North America, it is named after its similarity to the hazel tree. Witch hazel has woody stems, large leaves and spidery yellow flowers. Historically used to prevent internal bleeding, witch hazel extract is a useful astringent that also soothes the skin. It is one of the most widely used plants in Western medicine and the leaves contain high levels of a particular tannin, *hamamelitannin*, which gives them astringent properties and a healing action on veins. Tannins occur widely in nature and are used to heal the skin.

According to medical herbalism, tannins are responsible for binding a protein called *albumen* in the skin to form a tight layer which is resistant to disease. This separates the bacteria which have settled on the skin and protects against potential irritation.

Witch hazel lotion is made from the leaves and twigs of the plant and is readily available from most chemists. Although this contains only ten per cent tannins and up to fifteen per cent alcohol, it is a handy ingredient for homemade skin fresheners, especially for inflamed skin conditions, compresses to heal wounds and soothing face masks.

Witch hazel capsules are also prescribed for internal use by medical herbalists to treat problems with veins and capillaries, including varicose veins, piles and broken thread veins on the face. Compresses made from witch hazel are also an effective external remedy for haemorrhoids (piles).

Yarrow *Achillea millefolium*

A tall herb with attractive feathery foliage and white flowers, yarrow gets its name from the Latin for 'thousand-leaf'. It is also known as the healing herb, as it helps other plants nearby resist attacks from disease and pests. Yarrow has astringent properties and is useful for pepping up a poor circulation and for improving skin tone. It also contains azulene, the skin soother found in some other herbs, notably chamomile. Culpeper used yarrow to prevent hair loss and modern herbalists regard yarrow as a useful all-round tonic that can also help to lower blood pressure. It may be prescribed to help menstrual problems such as unusually heavy periods. Yarrow tea can also be used to help ease colds and influenza. Externally, an infusion of yarrow leaves and flowers can be used as an effective skin tonic, and is useful for soothing sore skin conditions. It is also efficient at promoting wound healing and improving the skin's own micro-circulation.

ESSENTIAL OILS

In addition to plant extracts made from flowers, leaves and roots, many botanicals also contain essential oils which are remarkably effective in beauty recipes. Essential oils can be defined in two ways: their scientific explanation is that many plants contain high concentrations of volatile oils which give plants their distinctive flavours and aromas. These aromatic, essential or volatile oils are made up from a wide variety of different chemical constituents. A single essential oil may contain as many as fifty individual ingredients, including substances such as *phenol, carvacrol, linalol* and *geraniol*. Aromatherapists, who use essential oils for therapeutic massage, are more likely to adopt a less clinical approach when it comes to defining essential oils. They often describe them as the 'life force' or 'soul' of the plant and believe that each essential oil has different characteristics and uses. Whether you take the more pragmatic and analytical approach, or prefer to follow the folklore, there is no doubt that essential oils can be extremely useful in caring for the body and encouraging well-being.

Essential oils can be extracted from plants in two main ways – by using either steam or solvent distillation. Steam distillation involves placing the plant material in a flask, heating to a high temperature and collecting the steam. As the steam cools and turns back into water, the essential oil from the plant floats to the surface where it can be collected. Steam distillation is the best method for extracting pure essential oils and most of the expensive varieties are extracted this way. The other method of solvent extraction involves placing the plant material in a flask and mixing with a chemical solvent such as *hexane*. The mixture is stirred and heated to release the essential oils from the plant before the solvent is evaporated away. Solvent extraction is common in the perfume industry, where natural flower fragrances are still used by some of the more expensive brands. However, it is not the best method for producing essential oils for skincare as traces of the solvent are always left behind in the oil. Technically, anything that has been produced by solvent extraction should be called an 'absolute' and not an 'essential' oil. Common examples include rose absolute or jasmine absolute, which are extremely rare to find as essential oils made by steam distillation.

The main problem when buying essential oils is knowing exactly what is inside the bottle. Always look for the words 'pure essential oil', on the label which mean that the oil has not been diluted with a cheaper vegetable oil before bottling. Some oils are sold as 'aromatherapy oils' or 'fragrance oils' and should not be confused with genuine, highly concentrated essential oils. Most healthfood shops stock reputable ranges and there is also a list of reliable mail-order suppliers at the back of the book. Another safety check is to make sure that your supplier is registered with EOTA (the Essential Oil Trade Association) as their members are regularly checked for quality control. If in doubt, go by the price. Essential oils are not cheap and in most cases you do get what you pay for. However, because they are only used in tiny amounts, a good-quality essential oil will last a long time if kept cool and dark, and most oils have many health and beauty uses. All essential oils are naturally antiseptic and many are also naturally antibiotic. Some even help to boost the immune system and fight off bacterial, viral and fungal infections.

Aromatherapy

Aromatherapy is the art of using these essential oils mixed in a base or 'carrier' oil, such as almond or grapeseed oil, combined with massage. Aromatherapy works by releasing the aroma of these oils into the atmosphere where they are taken up by the nerve endings in the nose and relayed to the brain. Here they can have a powerful effect on mood, emotions and mental states. Essential or volatile oils also have a very small molecular structure enabling them to slip through the surface of the skin and end up in the bloodstream. This is why the oils used on the skin in massage can be so effective in treating not only skin complaints but also disorders as diverse as hormonal problems and cellulite.

Because essential oils end up circulating in the bloodstream, it is wise to use caution if using them during pregnancy. Stimulating herb and spice oils should be avoided and replaced with gentler oils such as chamomile, sandalwood, geranium and lemon (see overleaf). While small amounts of almost any oil are quite safe, for regular use it is best to consult a professional aromatherapist for personal advice during pregnancy. Pregnant or not, all essential oils are highly concentrated and should only ever be used in small quantities and always diluted either in a carrier oil or cream, or diffused in a warm bath. The only exceptions to this rule are when using lavender oil neat on burns, or dabbing small amounts of tea tree oil on to spots and pimples.

Essential oils to avoid during pregnancy

Aniseed, bay, basil, cassia, clary sage, cedarwood, clove, coriander, cinnamon, cypress, eucalyptus, hyssop, juniper, lemongrass, nutmeg, sage, savory, thyme, marjoram (including sweet marjoram), myrrh, pennyroyal, pine, rosemary, tansy, tea tree, wintergreen and wormwood.

Essential oils recommended during pregnancy

Citrus oils (e.g., mandarin, tangerine, bergamot and lemon), sandalwood, neroli, jasmine, geranium and chamomile. After the first three months, lavender, rose and melissa may also be used in moderation.

Essentially Beautiful

The best essential oils for beauty recipes are listed in alphabetical order below, together with their main uses. It is not necessary to buy all the oils at once, simply start with a couple of the most commonly used ones such as lavender and geranium. It may be more economical to share essential oils with a friend, or to buy them direct from a local aromatherapist who can supply smaller quantities to experiment with.

Bergamot *Citrus bergamia*

The bergamot is a cross between an orange and a lemon and grows in northern Italy around the area of Bergamo, which gave the fruit its name. The essential oil is extracted from the oil-bearing glands on the surface of the fruit. It has a sweet, citrus smell and is used to flavour Earl Grey tea, and is a traditional ingredient in eau de cologne. The uplifting, refreshing scent of bergamot oil is useful for adding to a reviving bath and is the perfect solution for lifting the spirits after a tiring day. Bergamot suits combination and oily skintypes but as with all citrus oils, should not be used in the sun or before going on a sunbed. This is because citrus oils contain substances that can photo-sensitise the skin in strong sunlight and may cause allergies.

Chamomile *Chamomilla matricara*

This essential oil comes from the flowers of this European herb. There are two main types of chamomile essential oil, Roman chamomile and German chamomile, and both are useful in skincare. However, it is the German variety (*Chamomilla matricara*) that is highly prized and more expensive. Chamomile oil has soothing, relaxing and calming properties and is safe to use on small children and during pregnancy. Both types of chamomile oil suit dry, sensitive and easily irritated skintypes and it is one of the few essential oils that can be used on inflamed skin conditions such as eczema.

Cypress *Cupressus sempervirens*

This essential oil is extracted from the leaves and twigs of the evergreen cypress tree. Its smell is similar to pine, although slightly sweeter and less overpowering. It is a useful oil in bodycare as it stimulates the circulation and can be used to treat water retention. Cypress is often added to anti-cellulite remedies and is excellent for improving over-all skin tone. It is mildly astringent and is best suited to normal, combination and oily skintypes. Cypress oil can also be added to a warm bath to stimulate and revive aching muscles after exercise.

Eucalyptus *Eucalyptus globulus*

Native to Australia where eucalyptus shoots are the favourite food of koala bears, the essential oil comes from the leaves and twigs of this tall tree. Eucalyptus is a powerful and un-mistakably pungent oil widely used in cough mixtures and bronchial expectorants. The essential oil is naturally anti-biotic and anti-inflammatory and therefore has a wide range of medicinal uses. In skincare it is excellent for healing spots, boils and pimples and may be dabbed neat in tiny quantities on to the affected area.

Eucalyptus oil is also useful as a burning essence to ease the stuffiness of nasal congestion. Two or three drops in a bowl of hot water also makes an instant invigorating steam inhalation. Eucalyptus oil has high levels of camphor, which is an irritant, and is therefore unsuitable for use on the skin of babies and children under the age of two. It is also too strong to use in most facial recipes but one drop mixed with a dessertspoonful of jojoba oil is a useful antiseptic massage oil for spotty backs and complexions.

Fennel *Foeniculum vulgare*

The seeds of the fennel flower are crushed to produce this essential oil, which is a useful diuretic and good for cases of water retention. Only the essential oil known as 'sweet fennel' should be used on the body and this is traditionally associated with female reproductive organs. Although fennel oil is best avoided during pregnancy, a few drops mixed with almond oil are often helpful for massage during breastfeed-ing as it can help to increase the milk supply. Sweet fennel has a faintly aniseed scent and is most often included in skin-care to tone puffy and slackened skin tissues.

Frankincense *Boswellia carterii*

This essential oil dates back to Biblical times and beyond, when it was burned as incense in temples. The oil comes from the gummy resin produced by a tree that is native to Somalia in Africa. Frankincense has a purifying and toning action on the skin and is especially useful in anti-wrinkle remedies. Used sparingly, it can be added to night creams and neck lotions to help deter fine lines and wrinkles by stim-ulating skin cells. Perhaps because of its association with churches, the aroma of frankincense also has a calming effect when inhaled and is a useful burning oil for times under pressure or if we need greater mental concentration. Massaging a few drops into the temples and scalp is also a quick and easy way to clear the mind and reduce tension headaches.

Geranium *Pelargonium graveolens*

There are several hundred different varieties of geranium but only a few are used to make the sweet-smelling essential oils. Among the best is rose geranium, which is extracted from a variety of geranium leaves that smell just like roses, and this is an exceptionally good oil for adding to skincare recipes. It is also a good option for adding a rose fragrance to recipes at a fraction of the cost of pure rose oil. All geranium essential oils have a toning and soothing action on the skin and suit most skintypes, including dry and sensitive complexions. They also have a normalising action on the skin and are good for balancing a combination complexion and for combatting cellulite.

In addition to rose geranium, there are other types of geranium oils that may be used in recipes which have a variety of sweet, floral fragrancs. However, all should be used sparingly as it is easy to overdo the amount needed and end up with a sickly sweet scent.

Ginger *Zingiber officinale*

This essential oil is extracted from the roots or rhizome of this traditional Chinese herb. Used for thousands of years to ward off coughs, colds and general infections, ginger oil is a powerful antiseptic and has a warming action on the body. It should be used with caution in skincare as it is extremely potent and can easily irritate sensitive complexions. However, ginger oil is useful for boosting the blood supply to the surface of the skin and can help complaints such as chilblains, rheumatism and muscular aches and pains. It is also a perfect ingredient for making warming footbaths, if you are suffering from a cold or influenza.

Jasmine *Jasminum officinale*

Pure jasmine essential oil from Grasse in the South of France is one of the most expensive natural skincare ingredients. It comes from the tiny white flowers which must be picked by hand each morning before the sun rises high in the sky and evaporates their oil content. The scent of the jasmine flowers is so strong that it fills the hillsides in Grasse during the traditional harvest months of September and October. Once the flowers have been collected, the oil is extracted using solvents to make a jasmine absolute (steam-distilled jasmine oil is extremely rare). The smell of jasmine is extremely sweet and over-powering if used in excess. It is a costly ingredient, but a little goes a very long way and one small bottle will last several years if stored in a cool, dark place. Jasmine oil is traditionally associated with femininity and has uplifting properties. One drop will luxuriously fragrance a warm bath and leave a lingering aroma on the skin. Jasmine oil suits all skintypes, especially delicate skins and is reputed to improve the appearance of stretchmarks and scar tissue.

Juniper berry *Juniperus communis*

This essential oil comes from the dark, ripe berries of the prickly juniper bush that grows wild throughout Southern Europe. The oil has a distinctively pungent and slightly bitter aroma that is used by distillers to flavour gin. It is also used in perfumery and often added to macho-smelling male aftershaves. Juniper essential oil has anti-fungal properties and is also a powerful diuretic. This is why it is often added to lotions and oils that help treat cellulite, and puffiness due to fluid retention. However, it has a powerful effect on the skin and should be used sparingly. In skincare, juniper oil suits combination and oily skintypes and can be used in facial oils to treat acne.

Lavender *Lavendula officinalis*

This is the king of essential oils and an essential part of all health and beauty routines. It is extracted from the flowering spikes of the lavender plant and there are many different varieties. The best is from *Lavendula officinalis* and this, of course, is also the most expensive. Spike lavender, or *Lavendula spica*, is another variety that is also popular with aromatherapists. By crossing these two varieties of lavender, botanists have produced a similar plant called *lavendin*. This hybrid plant is much easier to grow and produces many more flowering spikes and so its essential oil is quite a bit cheaper than pure lavender oil. As an example, lavender produces around fifteen to twenty kilos of essential oil per hectare, while lavendin produces between eighty to 120 kilos per hectare. Not surprisingly, there is a temptation for less scrupulous suppliers to sell lavendin incorrectly labelled as the more expensive pure lavender oil. However, lavendin does have a lovely smell and is widely used in the perfume industry and by toiletry manufacturers to disguise the smell of harsh detergents.

Pure, neat lavender oil can be used on burns (worth keeping some in the kitchen) and rapidly heals scar tissues. It is also used to treat headaches, including migraine, stress and insomnia. It is gentler on the skin and more effective at healing open wounds than modern antiseptics and is definitely an essential oil for the first-aid box. Lavender oil also has many other uses and is a versatile ingredient in many skincare recipes. It has fortifying, balancing and toning properties, as well as being naturally antibiotic and anti-fungal. It suits most skintypes except very dry, sensitive complexions and is an excellent oil for the bath and general massage blends.

Lemon *Citrus limonum*

This essential oil is one of the easiest to extract as it comes from the oil-laden glands on the fruit's skin. This means it is also one of the cheapest essential oils to buy. Lemon oil has many useful skincare properties as it is anti-fungal, diuretic and naturally stimulating. However, it should not be used directly on the skin before going out into the sunshine as it contains ingredients that can react with ultra-violet light and cause skin sensitivity. Lemon oil is useful for adding to baths to pep up the circulation and revive the senses. It acts as an all-round tonic and is helpful for adding to skin fresheners, anti-cellulite creams and lotions for combination or oily skintypes.

Mandarin *Citrus nobilis*

This is another essential oil that is easily extracted from the rind of a citrus fruit. It has a sweet, subtle scent and is good for adding to children's baths and skincare routines. Mandarin oil is soothing, up-lifting and toning. It also helps improve the circulation and so is a good ingredient for many body oils and lotions. A few drops of mandarin oil also makes a reviving bath and it is useful for cases of insomnia and nervous tension. As with other citrus oils, it should not be used before exposing the skin to sunlight or before going on a sunbed. All citrus oils also have a limited shelf-life and should be used within one year of purchase.

Melissa *Melissa officinalis*

True melissa is extremely rare but it can be found – at a price! It is extracted from lemon balm leaves and has a powerful lemony fragrance (one or two drops added to a warm bath will not only fragrance the water but also the entire house). Most essential oil sold as melissa oil is an inferior blend of citrus oils and lemongrass. Look for the words *'Melissa officinalis'* on the label, or go by the price. As with most essential oils from reputable suppliers, you tend to get what you pay for.

Melissa oil was an important ingredient in the famous Melissa Water, one of the first commercial perfumes made in medieval times by Carmelite monks in Italy. Synthetic versions are still used in many modern perfumes and aftershaves and it is a versatile beauty oil. Melissa oil has soothing, uplifting and toning properties. It is one of the very best oils for adding to a reviving bath or massage oil blend. Pure melissa oil has also been found to help combat the *Herpes simplex* virus and its anti-viral activity has been proven in clinical trials. It suits all skintypes and adds a wonderfully fresh scent to lotions for the face and body.

Myrrh *Commiphora myrrha*

This unusual essential oil comes from the bark and resin of an African bush. Highly valued for thousands of years, myrrh was one of the original gifts given by the Magi to the infant Jesus. Myrrh is strongly antiseptic and has anti-fungal properties. It is not widely used in skincare because of its pungent aroma but is useful for healing the mouth and gums, and has valuable anti-inflammatory properties. It can also be used on ulcers and boils as it has an anti-microbial effect. Myrrh is best suited to normal, combination and oily skins but should always be used sparingly. It may be added to massage blends to soothe and strengthen the skin, and a few drops in the bath can help cases of candidiasis (thrush).

Neroli *Citrus aurantium*

This sweet-smelling oil comes from orange blossom and is a traditional skincare ingredient. It is also probably the most expensive essential oil you can buy. Neroli oil has a soft, fruity scent that is widely used in eau de cologne and general perfumery. The essential oil has uplifting and restorative properties and can help ease tension and relax the body. It also helps improve the skin's own micro-circulation and can help problem, spotty skins. Neroli is best suited to normal, combination and oily skintypes, although it can also be used for its fabulous fragrance alone in many beauty remedies.

Patchouli *Pogostemon patchouli*

An aromatic, distinctive oil that comes from the dried leaves of a Chinese herb, patchouli oil has been used as a natural perfume for thousands of years, especially in the Middle East and India, where it was regarded as a sacred herb. The essential oil has many skincare properties and is both antibiotic and anti-fungal. In addition, it has a toning, strengthening effect on the skin and can be diluted with wheatgerm oil and used to repair damaged skin and fade scar tissue. Patchouli is also helpful added to anti-cellulite creams and acts as a gentle skin toner. It may be used in hair and scalp remedies to treat hair loss and flaking scalp conditions. Alternatively, patchouli oil can be used simply to give a warm, spicy aroma to massage oil blends or added to a warm bath as an aromatic treat.

Peppermint *Mentha piperata*

The leaves, flowers and stalks of this common garden herb are used to make peppermint essential oil. Because of its naturally high menthol content peppermint feels cool and refreshing on the skin and is effective in invigorating skincare products such as foot lotion and after-sun creams. It may be added to baths to tone and stimulate the skin, but do not use more than a couple of drops otherwise it will make even the hottest bathwater feel cold against the skin. Peppermint is also useful for clearing the mind and encouraging productivity (the Japanese squirt it into the atmosphere in their factories as it has been proved to enhance output). Due to its high menthol content, peppermint oil is a common irritant and is not suitable for use on the skin of babies or children under two years of age. It should also be avoided by those with delicate or sensitive skins and is best suited to oilier complexions.

Pine *Pinus palustris*

This powerful antiseptic oil has many medicinal uses and is widely used in disinfectants and detergents. The essential oil is extracted from the needles and twigs of the American pine tree and has a pungent, distinctive smell. Pine oil is often too over-powering to use in beauty remedies, although it is useful for some scalp oils and as a topical antiseptic for spots and boils. It is a potent stimulant and a couple of drops in a warm bath will rev up the circulation and get the body glowing. Pine oil also helps to fight off infections and is a useful oil in steam inhalations for all kinds of nasal and respiratory complaints.

Rose *Rosa damascena*

As with jasmine oil, pure rose oil is rare and extremely expensive. Most pure rose oil is, in fact, a rose absolute produced by solvent extraction. It is extremely difficult for cosmetic chemists to copy the natural rose fragrance synthetically as it has over 500 different chemical constituents. Rose oil has fabulous skincare properties which is why it has been so highly prized throughout the centuries. It is also traditionally related to the female reproductive organs and has a soothing, calming effect on the skin. Aromatherapists may use rose oil to treat depression and hormonal problems including PMS. Rose oil is best suited to dry, fragile and more mature complexions and is also a good children's oil. It can be added to a warm bath for a luxuriant soak and is especially

good for pampering the body during the later stages of pregnancy. Rose oil is also used because of its exquisite smell and
can be added to scent skin creams and lotions. Less expensive alternatives with a similar fragrance include rose
geranium and rosewood.

Rosemary *Rosmarinus officinalis*

The flowering tops of this herb are used to extract the
strongly scented essential oil. One of the most antiseptic and
stimulating oils, rosemary also has diuretic properties. It also
has a high camphor content and should not be used on
babies or small children. Rosemary oil is a common ingredient in many fine fragrances and aftershaves, and has been
used in perfumery since 1370 when it was first included in
Hungary water. In other aspects of beauty culture it is a useful oil to add to hair and scalp blends as it helps relieve
itching, flaking scalp conditions and may even help combat
hair loss. Rosemary is also used in massage blends for stiff
joints and aching muscles and has mild painkilling properties. It suits combination and problem skins and can also be
used in treatments to improve the condition of cellulite and
loss of skin tone.

Rosewood *Aniba rosaeodora*

Also known as *rose de bois*, this essential oil smells like rose
petals although it actually comes from the bark of a South
American tree. Although rosewood has fewer skincare properties than pure rose oil, it is toning on the skin and has an
uplifting scent that can be used as a subtle fragrance in skin
creams. It is also useful in body massage blends and for
adding to a warm, reviving bath.

Sage *Salvia officinalis*

This powerful essential oil should be used with caution and
not at all during pregnancy. It is highly stimulating and antiseptic, and has many medicinal uses. It is best suited to
problem skins that benefit from its antibacterial properties
and it can also help in cases of dandruff and flaking scalps.
An important ingredient in herbal medicine, aromatherapists

also use sage oil to treat depression and severe menstrual or digestive disorders.

Sandalwood *Santalum album*

Made from the wood chippings of the sandalwood tree which is native to India, this essential oil has a distinctive, spicy aroma. It has a high alcohol content, making it highly antiseptic, and its aroma is also reputed to be an aphrodisiac. Sandalwood oil is a useful ingredient in many skincare remedies as it has a soothing and strengthening action on the skin. It is one of the gentlest oils to use in facial massage and can help soothe irritated and inflamed skin conditions. Sandalwood oil suits all skintypes and can even be used in treatments to help problem complexions including acne. A few drops added to a warm bath will transform it into a refreshing pick-me-up treatment, and the oil also adds a subtle aroma to massage blends and natural perfumes.

Sweet Marjoram *Origanum marjorana*

This essential oil is made from the flowering tops and leaves of the herb. There are several different types of marjoram and the closely related oregano oil, but only sweet marjoram should be used in skincare. Unfortunately, many of the cheaper essential oils on offer contain oregano or Spanish marjoram, which are far harsher on the skin. If in doubt, check that the oil is either *Origanum marjorana* or *Origanum hotensis*. It is strongly antiseptic and has calming, sedating properties that make it suitable for treating stress and insomnia (a few drops in a warm bedtime bath helps to relax the body and promote a good night's sleep). Sweet marjoram is also useful in massage blends designed to help sports injuries, muscular aches and sprains. Used in skincare, sweet marjoram suits oily and combination skintypes and is useful for dabbing neat on to spots and pimples.

Tea tree *Melaleuca alternifolia*

This increasingly popular oil comes from the leaves and twigs of an Australian tree. It has powerful antiseptic and anti-fungal properties, and is also anti-viral and naturally antibiotic, making it one of the most useful medicinal essential oils. It can be used to treat fungal infections such as candidiasis (thrush) and is several times more effective at killing germs than household disinfectant. First used by the Aborigines thousands of years ago, tea tree oil was issued in the first-aid kits of Australian soldiers in the Second World War. More recent trials by skin doctors have also shown that tea tree oil is effective at treating spotty, acne-prone skin and can be more helpful than many shop-bought preparations. For example, it is better at treating acne than benzoyl peroxide and yet has fewer skin damaging side-effects. Tea tree oil is best suited to oily and problem skins and may also be applied neat in small quantities to clear up spots and pimples. The essential oil is also useful for improving scalp disorders such as dandruff and a few drops may be added to shampoos and scalp lotions.

Thyme *Thymus vulgaris*

This is another highly medicinal essential oil that has been used for centuries for its powerfully antiseptic properties. It is made from the flowering tops of this common herb and has anti-viral and anti-fungal actions on the skin. A powerful healer, thyme oil must be used with caution and care on the skin. It is best suited to massage blends for sports injuries, arthritis and circulatory problems. It is useful in small doses to invigorate aching limbs and aromatherapists may also use the oil to help cases of high blood pressure or menstrual irregularity.

Ylang Ylang *Canang odorat*

The bright yellow flowers from a Madagascan tree produce this exotic essential oil which has a sweet smell that can be used as a cheaper alternative to jasmine oil. Ylang ylang has invigorating, uplifting properties and is best suited to normal and combination skintypes (it can occasionally irritate sensitive skins). The essential oil is also reputed to have an aphrodisiac effect and is certainly useful as a general tonic in times of stress. It can be used in skincare to add a subtle fragrance to many recipes and is also an excellent addition to reviving massage blends.

Fruits and vegetables

Most everyday fruits and vegetables make excellent ingredients for skincare. This is because they contain valuable enzymes that digest surface bacteria and leave the complexion glowing with good health. For best results, make sure the fruits or vegetables are as fresh as possible and free from dust and dirt. It is also worth choosing organically grown varieties where possible, as these do not contain traces of chemical pesticides, herbicides or fungicides that are best avoided on the skin.

Apple

There are over 1000 different varieties of apples and all are good sources of Vitamin C and the vegetable form of Vitamin A, beta carotene. Apples also contain minerals needed by the skin, including traces of potassium, calcium and magnesium. In addition, apples are a rich source of certain fruit acids, notably malic and tartaric acid which help to slough off dead cells from the skin's surface. They are useful ingredients in face masks and pure apple juice is an effective toner for combination complexions.

Avocado

This is technically a fruit because it contains a seed, although it is most often used in cooking savoury dishes. The avocado is one of nature's best beautifiers and contains all the ingredients needed to keep our skin cells healthy. It is naturally rich in plant oils that moisturise and smooth the skin. It also contains potassium, B Vitamins, beta carotene, Vitamin E and traces of iron. Avocados can be used on their own to make a moisturising face mask or added to hair conditioners and skin scrubs. The insides of the avocado skin are also good to rub over the body just before a shower as this dislodges dead skin cells and leaves the body feeling smooth.

Banana

The banana is nature's own convenience food and contains high levels of vitamins and minerals including potassium, magnesium, phosphorus, beta carotene, folic acid and Vitamin C. The sticky texture of mashed bananas also has many uses in natural beauty. Banana paste can be used as a skin-soothing face mask and also makes an excellent hair pack for dry, brittle hair.

Carrot

Carrots are rich in beta carotene, the skin-saving vitamin that gives some fruits and vegetables an orange or yellow colour. The main benefit of beta carotene is that it is an anti-oxidant, which means that it protects the skin from damage caused by free radical activity. This is a highly destructive process which occurs when particles of oxygen trigger a chain-reaction of cell damage within the body. The best way to use carrots in skincare is to soak grated carrot in a good quality vegetable oil for a few days. The oil may then be strained off and used as a basic massage oil or added to other skincare blends. Take care when using carrot oil though, because if the colour of the liquid is too dark, it can temporarily stain the skin orange.

Cucumber

Popular with the Ancient Greeks for its soothing and re-freshing properties, a strip or two of fresh cucumber placed over the eyes reduces puffiness and swelling. According to the seventeenth-century herbalist Culpeper, cucumber makes a good face wash for cleansing the skin and clearing the eyes. Although cucumber is mainly water it does contain traces of useful nutrients, including Vitamin C, potassium, silicon and sulphur. These are all needed to keep skin cells strong and healthy, and help maintain skin elasticity. Cucumber extract is often added to skincare as it has mildly astringent properties and can help calm skin irritations. If using the cucumber skin (which contains most of the plant's vitamins and minerals) be sure to use unwaxed varieties which have not been sprayed with fungicides.

Ginger

This spicy underground stem (or rhizome) is best used freshly grated from the root. Ginger is a powerful antiseptic and should only be used sparingly on the skin. It is also a potent stimulant and when added to a warm bath will invigorate the body and get the circulation going. Ginger root is used extensively in Chinese herbal medicine and is reputed to be an effective painkiller. It contains high levels of essential oils and medical trials have shown that these help to thin the blood, lower cholesterol levels and reduce the risk of heart disease.

Lemon

All citrus fruits are naturally rich in Vitamin C, which is required by the skin to make collagen. This is a type of protein that literally holds the skin together, and maintains flexibility and strength. Lemon rind is also full of natural essential oils and if you peel a lemon with your fingers you will see the tiny oil glands on the surface of the fruit burst open to release the fragrant oils. Lemon rind can be added to a warm bath to invigorate the body, but make sure the lemons are the unwaxed variety which have not been coated with chemical fungicides. Lemon juice is also useful as a mild form of natural acid, which helps soften hard water and dislodge detergent and soap residues from the skin.

Papaya

Also known as the paw-paw, papaya is a useful skincare ingredient because it contains the enzyme *papain*. This is a powerful fruit enzyme that digests protein and can be used on the skin to get rid of dead skin cells that can clog the pores and lead to spots. Papain has also been used by herbalists to help heal scar tissue and assist wound healing. The inside of papaya skins may be rubbed over the body before stepping into the shower and this is also a gentle way to shift dead skin cells that tend to accumulate on the upper arms, elbows, hips and thighs.

Pineapple

The pineapple contains another potent protein-digesting enzyme called *bromalin* which is also an excellent skin buffer. In Sri Lanka, women rub the insides of pineapples over their bodies to remove dead skin cells, and pineapple skin can also be used as the basis for a facial scrub. Fresh pineapple is the best type to use in skincare as the tinned variety has been heat treated and this destroys some of its natural enzymes. Pineapple is an excellent ingredient in face masks and treatments for spotty, problem complexions as it gently dissolves sebum and keeps the pores free from dirt and dead cell debris.

Potato

Potatoes are an excellent source of Vitamin C and have several uses in skincare. The juice from raw potatoes is a good skin soother and can be used to treat irritated and inflamed complexions. This can either be extracted using an electric vegetable juicer or may be bought in bottles from a healthfood shop. Slices of raw potato also make useful eye masks as they help counteract puffiness and reduce swelling. In addition, potatoes contain high levels of natural starch, and potato flour can be used in skincare recipes to thicken pastes and skin creams.

4

Cleansers and Skin Tonics

The starting point for a clear, glowing complexion is an efficient cleanser. One of the earliest recorded skin cleansers is cold cream. Originally invented by the Greek physician Galen, his recipe was based on beeswax, olive oil and rosewater. Cold cream gets its name because it is cooling on the skin and works as a cleanser when the oil and wax melt on to the face to loosen dirt, make-up and sebum. These can then be removed swiftly with tissues or a hot, damp facecloth to leave the skin feeling clean and soft. Modern versions of cold cream replace olive oil with cheaper mineral oil, and the beeswax is replaced with synthetic substitutes. However, the original cold cream is easy to make at home and is an excellent cleanser for very dry skin that is easily upset and irritated by washing with soap and water. This recipe has the sweet scent of honey and roses and is also a soothing skin moisturiser. In addition, it is useful as a baby's barrier cream, hand cream and rich, fragrant body cream.

Cold Cream Cleanser

20 g (¾ oz) beeswax
40 ml (8 tsp) olive oil
80 ml (3 fl oz) almond oil
½ tsp lecithin granules (or 3 lecithin capsules)
40 ml (8 tsp) rosewater
4 drops rose essential oil
(rosewood or rose geranium oils may be used instead)

This recipe involves melting the beeswax and vegetable oils in a double-boiler. A Pyrex jug is one of the easiest to use for this as it can be placed inside a larger saucepan with its handle hooked over the edge.

Place the beeswax, olive oil and almond oil in a small saucepan, jug or bowl and place this inside a larger pan that has been half filled with water. Bring the water to the boil, stirring the wax and oil mixture continuously. When the wax has completely melted, stir in the lecithin granules or snip the ends from the lecithin capsules and empty their contents into the mixture.

Remove from the heat and stir well until the lecithin has dissolved. Continue stirring while the mixture cools and add the rosewater.

Beat to a smooth paste and add the drops of essential oil and mix again. While the mixture is still soft, use a knife or spatula to transfer the cream into small, airtight jars. Scrape the sides of the container to remove all traces of the cream before it solidifies.

Simple soap and water are amongst the oldest type of skin cleansers and are still the number-one method of cleaning the skin throughout the world. Soap is an alkaline substance made from animal or vegetable fats, mixed with caustic soda and sodium salts for bars of soap, and potassium salts in liquid soaps. Soap was first documented by the Ancient Egyptians, who made it from the soapwort plant, which is characterised by its unusual ability to foam in water. Native to Asia and parts of Europe, the soapwort plant is an attractive plant with reddish, fragrant flowers and is still used as the basis of some of the more expensive vegetable soaps.

Most modern soaps are more likely to contain beef tallow mixed with vegetable fats, such as coconut oil and palm kernel oil, which help them lather.

Milled soaps are the most common as they are the quickest and easiest to manufacture. They contain the highest proportion of animal fats, are highly alkaline and produce the most lather. The so-called super-fatted soaps simply contain more oils or fats such as lanolin, olive oil or cocoa butter and are less likely to dry out the skin. However, all soaps tend to be strongly alkaline, with a pH value of between seven and ten. This can cause complexion problems because the surface of the skin is naturally acidic, with a pH value of 4.5 to 6.5. Washing with soap temporarily disrupts the delicate pH balance, disturbs the skin's natural oils and can lead to dryness and irritation.

Another problem with cleansing the face with soap is the washing water itself. Soap combines with the calcium and magnesium mineral deposits in hard water to leave an unattractive scum both around the rim of the basin and on your skin. This residue of soap suds can further dry and irritate the skin. Unless you live in a soft water area it is best to follow soap and water cleansing with a gentle skin tonic to remove any potentially irritating residues that remain.

Using soap to clean the face is really only a suitable option for those with combination or oily complexions. However, soap will not remove oil-based make-up, which is not soluble in water, so use a cream cleanser such as cold cream first. Medicated soaps can also cause problems when their antiseptic properties overly dry the skin. Side-effects of using medicated soaps on a regular basis include skin flaking, and mottling on the surface of coloured skins. They are also not particularly effective in combatting serious skin disorders such as acne. Ingredients commonly included in medicated soaps include salicylic acid, benzoyl peroxide and sulphur. If you like using a medicated soap or have an oily, spotty complexion, try the recipe for *Gently medicated soap* (page 80) that relies instead on gentler antiseptic ingredients such as lavender and tea tree essential oils.

Other types of soap include transparent or glycerine soaps. These contain higher proportions of coconut oil or castor oil and are usually more moisturising. After manufacture, glycerine soaps need to be stored for several weeks to harden before being wrapped. Because they take longer to manufacture they invariably cost more. They are also not very good at producing a lather and are better suited to more sensitive skins, although they do end up sticking to the bottom of the soap dish.

Stylish soaps that can be made at home include exfoliating bars that contain tiny granules of sand, oatmeal or wheatgerm. These work by gently dislodging dead skin cells as the soap is rubbed over the body, leaving the skin thoroughly invigorated and glowing.

Oatmeal and orange soap balls

275 g (10 oz) soft vegetable glycerine soap
50 g (2 oz) medium ground oatmeal
30 ml (6 tsp) almond oil
5 ml (1 tsp) finely grated orange zest
12 drops lemon essential oil

The key to adapting soaps to suit your own skintype is to start with a good quality soap as a base. Larger healthfood shops and herbal suppliers sell blocks of white vegetable glycerine soap which is the best to use. Most other soaps are triple milled which makes them difficult to work with (they also contain beef tallow, which smells terrible when melted). These old-fashioned soap balls contain oatmeal, which is mildly exfoliating and moisturising on the skin.

Prepare the soap by slicing or grating into small pieces. Place in a small saucepan and melt over a high heat. Stir in the oatmeal and almond oil and mix thoroughly.

Remove from the heat, stir in the grated orange zest and lemon essential oil and allow the mixture to cool slightly.

Divide the mixture into four equal-sized portions and roll each one into a small ball. Place the soap balls on a wire rack and leave overnight to harden. When the soaps have set hard, wrap in tissue paper and store in a cool, dry place.

Gently medicated soap

150 g (5 oz) soft olive oil soap
50 ml (2 fl oz) strong sage tea
10 drops tea tree essential oil
10 drops lavender essential oil
1 tsp almond oil or jojoba oil (to grease moulds)

An excellent cleansing bar to use on oily, combination or acne-prone complexions. The essential oils purify the skin and have a gentler effect than many commercial soaps.

Make the sage tea by infusing a dessertspoonful (10 ml) of dried sage in a cup of almost boiling water. While this is steeping, prepare the soap by chopping or grating into small pieces. I find this recipe works best using the blocks of green olive oil soap from Marseille, which can be found in health-food shops and some chemists.

Place the soap pieces in a small saucepan and begin to melt over a high heat. Add the sage tea and stir thoroughly. Remove from the heat and allow to cool before adding the essential oils, as heat reduces their potency.

Pour the soap mixture into greased moulds (such as small bun tins, china ramekins or egg cups) and leave in a cool place to harden overnight. Remove from the moulds using a sharp knife and wrap in tissue paper until ready to use.

Richly moisturising soap

150 g (5 oz) good quality, unperfumed soap
15 ml (1 tbsp) coconut oil
50 ml (2 fl oz) strong chamomile tea
10 ml (2 tsp) olive oil
5 ml (1 tsp) honey
5 drops sandalwood or geranium essential oil
5 ml (1 tsp) almond or olive oil (to grease moulds)

Unlike many commercial soaps, this bar cleanses the skin thoroughly yet gently and leaves the skin feeling soft. It is gentle enough to use on babies' and children's sensitive skins.

Make the chamomile tea by infusing a dessertspoon (10 ml)

of dried chamomile flowers, or one herb tea bag, in a cup of almost boiling water. While this is steeping, prepare the soap as above and melt in a small saucepan together with the coconut oil over a high heat.

Add the chamomile tea, olive oil and honey. Mix thoroughly and allow to cool. Add the sandalwood or geranium essential oils to fragrance the soap (or substitute your own favourite essence). Pour the mixture into pre-prepared moulds as before and leave overnight in a cool place to harden.

Simple soapwort cleanser

10 g (¼ oz) finely chopped soapwort root
600 ml (1 pint) water
45 ml (3 tbsp) rosewater (optional)

Although it looks like cold tea and smells a bit strange, this is the simplest cleanser to make and works well on sensitive skins. It is also useful if you live in a hard water area, as regular soaps often react with the alkaline mineral deposits in the water and leave a scum on the skin. Soapwort root is available from good herbal suppliers.

Place the chopped soapwort root in a small saucepan and pour on the water. Bring to the boil, turn the heat down, cover and simmer on a low heat for 15–20 minutes. This mixture gives off a 'farm yard' smell while simmering, which can be disguised by adding the optional rosewater.

Remove the pan from the heat and allow the mixture to cool. Strain the mixture through a coffee filter to remove the soapwort pieces and bottle the remaining liquid. To use, pour a small amount into the palm of the hand, massage into skin and rinse with plenty of warm water.

Chamomile cleanser

85 ml (3 fl oz) almond oil
40 g (1½ oz) cocoa butter
10 drops chamomile essential oil

This rich cleanser is an excellent make-up remover and even shifts stubborn waterproof mascara. It is suitable for all skin-types, including dry and sensitive. It is also good for oily complexions as the oils in the cream dissolve the skin's own sebum and remove grease from the surface of the skin.

First, melt the cocoa butter in a small saucepan over a low heat. Remove from the stove and stir in the almond oil. Whisk in the chamomile essential oil and stir well. Pour the mixture into a clean, airtight jar.

To use, rub a small amount of the cleansing cream into the face and neck, massaging in gentle circular movements with the fingertips. Remove with a clean cotton cloth, such as a baby's muslin, or soft face flannel wrung out in hot water. Rinse the cloth and repeat until all traces of the cleanser have been removed.

Dip the cloth into cold water and pat over the face and neck to tighten the skin. Used regularly, this cleanser will help to soften and remove blackheads and can be used around the nose and chin twice a day to keep the skin clear.

Kaolin cleanser

5 ml (1 tsp) Fuller's earth
15 ml (1 tbsp) warm water
5 ml (1 tsp) finely ground oatmeal
2 drops lavender or geranium essential oil

This is a good cleanser for oily, combination and acne-prone skins. Combine the Fuller's earth powder with the warm water and mix to a smooth paste. Stir in the oatmeal and lavender or geranium essential oil.

To use, pin hair back from the face and apply to the skin using the fingertips, or a clean facial sponge. Allow to dry on the skin for one minute before rinsing off, using gentle massaging movements and plenty of warm rinsing wter. Remove any residues of cleanser with the *Floral skin freshener* (see page 84) for oily skins.

Honey purifier

5 ml (1 tsp) honey
250 ml (8 fl oz) hot water

Honey is naturally antiseptic and moisturising. This simple treatment is effective for all skintypes and can be carried out once a week to help keep the complexion clear.

Start by rubbing the honey into the face using small circular movements (runny honey is the easiest to use).

Dip the fingertips into the cup of hot water and repeat. The heat from the water will encourage the skin to soften and help shift embedded dirt and debris. After a few minutes of massage, rinse the face in clean, tepid water and pat dry.

Floral skin fresheners

150 ml (6 fl oz) fizzy (carbonated) mineral water
5 ml (1 tsp) cider vinegar
normal skins: 3 drops lavender + 3 drops geranium
    essential oils
dry skins: 3 drops sandalwood + 3 drops chamomile
    essential oils
oily skins: 3 drops lemon + 3 drops lavender essential oils

These floral waters are wonderfully refreshing on the face and are simple to tailor to your skintype. Unlike synthetic skin tonics they do not contain potentially irritating colourants, fragrances or preservatives.

First, measure the mineral water and cider vinegar into a screw-top bottle or jar and add the appropriate essential oils drop by drop. Replace the top of the container and shake well to mix the oils. Apply with cotton wool to remove traces of cleanser from the face.

Invigorating skin tonic

100 ml (4 fl oz) witch hazel
50 ml (2 fl oz) rosewater
2 drops rose essential oil (or rose geranium or rosewood)

Witch hazel has a pore-shrinking ability, due to the natural tannins found in the *Hamamelis* plant. These tannins are also found in nettles, and nettle tea may be used instead of witch hazel if desired. Both varieties are excellent for toning normal, combination and oily skins.

Place the ingredients in a screw-top bottle or jar and shake well. Use as a skin tonic to remove all traces of cleanser or soap-sud residues from the face and neck.

Alum astringent

250 ml (8 fl oz) warm water
5 ml (1 tsp) alum crystals
120 ml (4 fl oz) witch hazel

A true astringent contracts skin tissues, so if you dab a bit on the end of your tongue it will not only taste bitter but you should also feel the skin pucker. The astringent skin tonic is highly effective and can be made for a fraction of the price of shop-bought lotions. Alum is a form of aluminium crystals and can be found in chemists.

Dissolve the alum in the water, add the witch hazel and mix well. Store in a screw-top bottle or jar, away from heat and light.

Spotty skin tonic

100 ml (4 fl oz) witch hazel
10 ml (2 tsp) freshly squeezed lemon juice
2 drops tea tree essential oil
1 drop lemon essential oil

The fresh lemon juice used in this contains seven per cent citric acid which helps the pores appear smaller by puffing up the skin that surrounds them.

To make, simply measure all the ingredients into a screw-top bottle or jar. Shake well to mix the oils.

To use, apply with cotton wool and gently sweep over the skin, avoiding the eye area.

Extremely gentle skin freshener

100 ml (4 fl oz) rosewater
100 ml (4 fl oz) chamomile tea
2 drops sandalwood essential oil

Beware of commercial skin toners if your skin is dry or sensitive as they can contain high levels of alcohol to evaporate the liquid from the skin. Even alcohol-free varieties contain other chemicals to achieve the same effect, and rob the skin of valuable moisture.

Make the chamomile tea by infusing 1 dessertspoonful (10 ml) of dried chamomile flowers or 1 chamomile tea bag in a cup of almost boiling water. Allow to cool and strain.

Pour into a screw-top bottle or jar, add the rosewater and sandalwood essential oil and shake well to mix. Keep tightly sealed in a cool place, preferably in the fridge, and use within one week.

Barley skin freshener

75 g (3 oz) pot barley
750 ml (1¼ pints) water
4 drops lemon essential oil

This skin freshener is suitable for normal and combination complexions. It is based on barley water, which is a rich source of many minerals needed by the skin, including potassium, zinc and sulphur.

Place the pot barley and the water in a saucepan and bring to the boil. Cover and simmer on a low heat for 30 minutes, or until the barley has cooked through. Strain the liquid and transfer to a screw-top bottle or jar (the pearl barley may be kept and added to soups or stews).

Add the essential oil and shake well. Keep in the fridge and use after cleansing the face to refresh the skin.

Refreshing spritzer

100 ml (4 fl oz) fizzy (carbonated) mineral water
2 drops peppermint essential oil
3 drops neroli essential oil

Place all the ingredients in a screw-top bottle or jar and shake well. Transfer the liquid to a plastic spray bottle with a fine mist pump (available from chemists and good department stores).

Store in the fridge and use to lightly spritz over the face and neck.

This instant skin refresher is especially useful during hot weather and can also be sprayed over foundation and powder to set it in place.

5

Problem Solvers and Skin Savers

All skintypes benefit from a special treatment once in a while. Face masks and skin scrubs are the fastest way to get the complexion glowing, and they are quick and easy to make. The following recipes are split into sections according to skintype, and at the end of this chapter you will also find advice and treatments for more serious skin disorders, including acne, psoriasis and eczema.

Herbal steams

15 ml (1 tbsp) fresh or dried herb mixture as follows:
Normal skins: lavender and sage
Dry skins: chamomile and basil
Oily/Combination skins: mint and lemon peel
Bowl or basin of hot water
Large towel

A weekly herbal steam is a useful skin treatment for all skin-types. It is suitable for dry and sensitive complexions as the moisture from the steam helps plump up dehydrated skin cells. It is also a good treatment for oily and combination skins, as the heat from the steam gently softens blackheads or hardened plugs of sebum that can clog the pores and cause spots.

Simply fill a basin or large bowl with water which has been boiled and cooled slightly. Stir in the herbs and allow to infuse for a few minutes (you can use herbal tea bags if fresh or dried herbs are not available).

Place a large towel around your head and neck so that it forms a tent and lean over the bowl. Close the eyes and allow the steam to work on the skin for 1–3 minutes. Do not have the water so hot that the steam scalds the skin – a gentle heat is all that is required.

Afterwards, pat the skin dry with a cool, clean face cloth and apply a light moisturiser.

Re-moisturising mask

15 ml (1 tbsp) buttermilk or plain, live yoghurt
1 egg yolk
2.5 ml (½ tsp) honey
5 ml (1 tsp) mayonnaise

This richly moisturising mask contains natural lecithin from the egg yolk, which helps lock moisture into the skin. In addition, the buttermilk or yoghurt contains lactic acid which is also an excellent moisturiser and with regular use can help fade brown 'age' spots.

Mix all the ingredients together in a bowl until they form a smooth paste. Apply to clean, dry skin on the face and neck and leave for 15–20 minutes. Rinse thoroughly with plenty of warm water and pat dry.

A simpler version of this emollient mask may be made by mixing 2.5 ml (½ tsp) honey with one egg yolk. The honey forms a moisturising film on the face while the lecithin in the egg yolk is also deeply nourishing and helps bind moisture on to the skin's surface.

Oatmeal and mint refresher

60 ml (4 tbsp) finely ground oatmeal
50 ml (2 fl oz) hot water
15 ml (1 tbsp) fresh mint leaves

This fragrant face mask contains fresh peppermint to pep up the skin, and oatmeal to soothe minor irritations.

Mix the oatmeal with the water until it forms a thick paste. Wash and finely chop the mint leaves and add to the oatmeal. Leave for a few minutes for oatmeal to absorb the water and peppermint extracts before applying to freshly cleansed skin on the face and neck.

Relax for 20 minutes before rinsing away with warm water. Gently pat the skin dry and apply a light moisturiser.

Queen Victoria's face pack

50 g (2 oz) barley flour or brown rice flour
25 g (1 oz) runny honey
1 egg white

This recipe is similar to one used by the Royal Court during Queen Victoria's reign. It is excellent for refining and moisturising the complexion while tightening slack skin tissues.

In a small bowl, mix the flour with the runny honey until the mixture forms a stiff paste. Lightly beat the egg white and fold into the mixture.

Smooth on to clean skin on the face and neck. Relax for 15–20 minutes before rinsing with cool water. Gently pat the skin dry and apply a light moisturiser.

Banana skin pack

1 small ripe banana
25 g (1 oz) finely ground oatmeal
5 ml (1 tsp) runny honey

This face mask is excellent for re-moisturising tired, dehydrated skins. It also brings a bloom to tired, sallow or grey complexions.

Mash the banana in a small bowl until it forms a smooth paste. Stir in the finely ground oatmeal and runny honey. Mix well before applying to freshly cleansed skin on the face and neck.

Relax for 15–20 minutes before rinsing off using warm water. Pat the skin dry with a soft towel and apply a light moisturising cream.

Combination skin mask

15 ml (1 tbsp) finely ground oatmeal
15 ml (1 tbsp) live, plain yoghurt
½ freshly grated apple
10 ml (2 tsp) fresh lemon juice

A good facial mask to use for combination skins as the enzymatic action of the fresh apple and lemon juice helps tighten pores and also acts as a gentle exfoliant, dislodging dead skin cells and removing the build-up of sebum.

Mix the oatmeal with the plain yoghurt to form a paste. Add the freshly grated apple and lemon juice and stir well.

Apply to clean, dry skin on the face and neck. Relax for 15–20 minutes before rinsing thoroughly with warm water and patting the skin dry.

This mask is especially useful for slightly irritated or blotchy skins, as the oatmeal has a soothing effect. Make sure the live yoghurt contains *acidophilus*, as this type of beneficial bacterium is the most useful when it comes to clearing up spots and pimples.

Open-pore tightener

10 ml (2 tsp) Fuller's earth
10 ml (2 tsp) witch hazel
1 egg white, lightly beaten

This simple face mask is a fantastic skin tightener and re-duces the appearance of open pores. It will also absorb excess sebum and help unclog blocked pores.

Mix the Fuller's earth powder with the witch hazel to form a smooth paste. Add the lightly beaten egg white and stir vigorously to mix thoroughly.

Paint on to the face using a clean pastry brush or make-up brush. Apply several layers to the nose, chin and forehead, but avoid the immediate eye area and lips.

Leave for 5–10 minutes before rinsing thoroughly with plenty of cool water.

Our skin is constantly changing as fresh, young cells are formed to replace dead cells on the skin's surface. As the older skin cells die off they can easily clog the pores and lead to a dull, sallow-looking complexion. Exfoliation is the term given to any type of treatment that gently removes the top layer of dead skin cells, such as a skin scrub. Other kinds of effective exfoliators include soaps with gritty granules, facial brushes, abrasive creams, flannels, loofahs and even clay-based face masks that dislodge dead cells and remove them from the skin. An exfoliating treatment should always be ex-tremely gentle – if you are too zealous you may end up with a face full of broken veins.

Young skins can use a scrub twice a week to keep the com-plexion clear of blemishes, while more mature skins should stick to a once-weekly treatment. However, older skins do benefit from exfoliation, as it also helps speed up the rate at which fresh, young skin cells are replaced and this leads to a younger-looking complexion. Always avoid the fragile eye area, though, and be sure to apply a moisturiser after each treatment.

Dingy skin scrub

15 ml (1 tbsp) medium ground oatmeal
30 ml (2 tbsp) rose water
1 tsp granulated sugar
1 tsp honey

This is an excellent weekly treatment to brighten and refine all skintypes. The oatmeal helps soothe the skin while the sugar buffs away dead skin cells and also has an anti-bacterial effect.

Mix all the ingredients together in a bowl until they form a gritty paste. Apply to clean skin using gentle circular movements with the fingertips.

Concentrate on the nostrils, chin and forehead to dislodge dead skin cells and unclog the pores. Take care not to rub too hard, the smallest amount of pressure is all that is needed to dislodge flakes of dry, dingy-looking skin. Rinse with plenty of tepid water and pat the skin dry.

Instant exfoliator

1 ripe papaya

This type of skin exfoliation works by the enzymatic action of the papain found in the papaya fruit. Papain is able to dissolve dead keratin, the hardened protein found in dead skin cells. Instead of using granules such as sugar or oatmeal to buff the skin, this treatment relies on the papain to literally eat up the dead, dingy skin cells that make the skin look sallow and can lead to spots.

Simply slice the papaya fruit in half and peel away the skin in large pieces. Rub the inside of the skin over a freshly cleansed face and neck, massaging over the forehead, nose and chin for 1–2 minutes. Rinse the skin with clean, cool water and pat dry.

This treatment is good to use before a moisturising face mask as it takes off the dead surface cells so the face mask can penetrate the skin more easily.

Freckle fader

50 ml (2 fl oz) buttermilk
2.5 ml (½ tsp) freshly grated horseradish root
5 ml (2 tsp) lemon juice

Freckles are now considered to be extremely attractive, but if
you want to fade yours this lotion is worth trying. It also
works well on 'age' spots (also known as liver spots), that
often appear on the backs of the hands. However, for best
results the mixture should be applied daily for at least one
month and you must cover the area with a sunblock when
outdoors. If you can't get hold of buttermilk, you can substitute thin live yoghurt as this also contains lactic acid,
which is one of the active ingredients in this skin treatment.
Ready-grated horseradish root is available in jars from good
delicatessens and healthfood shops.

Combine the buttermilk, grated horseradish and lemon
juice and mix thoroughly. Apply to the affected parts only,
using a cotton but or cotton wool pad, as this lotion has
powerful skin bleaching properties. It is essential to avoid the
eye area and lips if using on the face, as the horseradish root
will sting and cause severe irritation.

Sensitive skin lotion

25 g (1 oz) dried marshmallow root
250 ml (8 fl oz) water

Marshmallow is an excellent skin-soothing herb and has
been used traditionally by herbalists for centuries to help
heal minor skin blemishes and irritations. Dried pieces of the
root are available from all good herbal suppliers.

Boil the water and pour over the marshmallow pieces.
Leave overnight to soak. Discard the pieces of root and pass
the liquid through a fine muslin cloth or paper coffee filter.

You should end up with approximately 90 ml (6 tbsp) of
rich, dark marshmallow extract.

Transfer the liquid to a clean screw-top bottle or jar. Apply
daily to the affected area using cotton wool. Store the lotion
in a cool, dark place such as the fridge.

Red-face compress

15 ml (1 tbsp) finely ground oatmeal
60 ml (4 tbsp) warm water
2 drops chamomile essential oil
piece of muslin cloth or flannel

This treatment is especially good for faces that redden easily or become blotchy and irritated in cold weather. Oatmeal helps shrink blood vessels and can help prevent tiny thread veins from forming.

Mix together the oatmeal and water and leave for a couple of minutes to thicken. Add the chamomile essential oil and stir well.

Dip the muslin cloth or flannel into the mixture and gently pat over the skin. Repeat several times.

Finally, place the compress over the face, lie down and relax for 15 minutes. Remove the compress, rinse out in clear, cool water and dab over the skin to remove any oatmeal residue. Pat the face and neck dry.

Puffy eye remedy

This treatment is simplicity itself and yet far more effective than any expensive eye gel. Simply rinse two strong tea bags (such as Darjeeling) under the tap and refrigerate for half an hour. Apply to clean eyelids and relax for 20 minutes before removing. The natural tannins in the tea leaves tighten the skin tissues around the eye area and dramatically reduce signs of puffiness and swelling.

Scar tissue lotion

15 ml (1 tbsp) rose hip oil
15 ml (1 tbsp) wheatgerm oil
3 drops sandalwood essential oil

Rose hip oil is a fabulous skin healer. It is available from good healthfood shops or from aromatherapy suppliers, and is sometimes sold under its Latin name of *Rosa rubiginosa*.

Measure the oils into a small bottle or jar and shake to mix. Rub on to the affected area twice daily. This lotion has a high Vitamin E content and is also a good treatment to help fade stretchmarks, or for use on surgical wounds once the stitches have been removed.

Herbal antiseptic lotion

10 g (¼ oz) marigold petals
10 g (¼ oz) golden seal, dried
10 g (¼ oz) pulsatilla, dried
100 ml (4 fl oz) water

Mix the dried herbs and flower petals together. Place in a small saucepan together with the water and simmer for 15 minutes. Leave to cool. Strain the lotion and apply the liquid to the affected area. This antiseptic lotion will keep in the fridge for several days.

Peppermint skin solution

5 ml (1 tsp) hazelnut or jojoba oil
1 drop peppermint essential oil

A useful treatment for spotty and acne-prone skins. Peppermint essential oil from *Mentha piperata* is the best variety to use as it contains a high proportion of natural plant hormones which can help this skin condition.

Mix 1 drop of essential oil in 5 ml (1 tsp) hazelnut oil and dab on to the affected area twice daily. Hazelnut or jojoba oils are the best carrier oils to use as they have excellent powers of penetration.

Tea tree spot-buster

5 ml (1 tsp) hazelnut or jojoba oil
2 drops tea tree essential oil
piece of muslin cloth or face flannel

An excellent treatment for stubborn spots on the face, neck and back. Before starting this treatment, it is essential to scrub the hands and nails thoroughly in soapy water. Then, rinse the muslin cloth or face flannel in clean hot water, wring out and apply to the area that needs treating.

When the cloth begins to cool, dip into hot water again, wring and repeat. The heat from the cloth gently softens spots, pimples and blackheads, dissolving the trapped sebum and releasing embedded grime.

Next, mix together the oils in the palm of one hand and apply to the affected area with warm fingertips. Massage gently to bring fresh blood supplies to the surface of the skin, which will help carry trapped toxins away from beneath the skin. Leave overnight.

Internal acne tonic

25 g (1 oz) blue flag
25 g (1 oz) echinacea
25 g (1 oz) cleavers
25 g (1 oz) figwort

Acne is caused by hormonal imbalances which can, in some cases, be linked to diet. One problem may be the body's ability to break down fats and carbohydrates, so the intake of saturated animal fats, sugar and refined carbohydrates should be strictly limited. Dietary supplements of zinc, beta carotene, cod liver oil and evening primrose oil can also be helpful. Medical herbalists have a high success rate for treating acne and this internal herbal tonic is also worth trying.

Blend the dried ingredients together and make up as an infusion by mixing 25 g (1 oz) of mixture to 600 ml (1 pint) of almost boiling water. Drink 3 small cupfuls daily after breakfast, lunch and dinner. The herbal extracts may be bought dried from a herbal supplier and made up daily.

Alternatively, a medical herbalist or herbal supplier can blend the mixture from liquid herbal tinctures. In this case, one 5 ml (1 tsp) spoonful should be taken three times a day after meals.

Eczema skin oil

15 ml (1 tbsp) calendula oil (see below)
15 ml (1 tbsp) St John's wort oil
5 ml (1 tsp) wheatgerm
5 ml (1 tsp) evening primrose oil

Eczema is now the most common childhood ailment in the western world and, unfortunately, appears to be on the increase. Those with eczema should avoid using soap or any kind of foaming detergent-baked cleanser on their skin. Cleansing oils from the chemist are a good option, as is this recipe for a topical treatment.

Mix all the oils together and store in an airtight jar away from heat and light. This richly nourishing oil contains important essential fatty acids, Vitamin E and several soothing herbal compounds to help relieve the itch and scaling associated with eczema. It is safe to use on babies and children and should be applied to clean, dry skin twice daily.

Evening primrose oil can be bought in a dropper bottle or obtained by squeezing out the contents from a couple of capsules. You can buy the calendula oil and St John's wort oil readymade from herbal or aromatherapy suppliers. Alternatively, make your own as follows in the recipe below.

Herbal oils

Many useful skin oils such as calendula oil (from pot marigold petals) and St John's wort oil may be made by macerating the flowers in a pure vegetable oil. Collect together the plant material and mix 15 ml (1 tbsp) of petals with 30 ml (2 tbsp) good-quality olive or almond oil.

Stir well, seal tightly and leave in a cool, dark place for 2–3 weeks. After this time, the healing extracts from the oil sacs on the petals will have been absorbed into the oil and the mixture can be strained and re-bottled ready for use in remedies.

Internal eczema tonic

25 g (1 oz) burdock root
25 g (1 oz) dandelion root
25 g (1 oz) yellow dock root
25 g (1 oz) dried nettles

Eczema is usually due to an internal disorder, so it is worth looking within for the actual cause. A dairy-free diet often helps, so substitute soya milk for cow's milk and avoid cream and cheese (although yoghurt and sheep's milk are tolerated by most eczema patients). Food additives, especially coal-tar food dyes, should also be avoided. Some types of eczema are also thought to be due to an essential fatty acid deficiency, so try taking a daily supplement of evening primrose oil. This can be especially helpful for babies and children. Herbal tonics, such as the recipes given below may also help, but be prepared for the symptoms to worsen initially before seeing a marked improvement.

Mix the dried ingredients together and make an infusion by combining 25 g (1 oz) of mixture to 600 ml (1 pint) of almost-boiling water.

Drink 3 small cupfuls daily after breakfast, lunch and dinner. The herbal extracts may be bought dried from a herbal supplier and made up daily. Alternatively, a medical herbalist or herbal supplier can blend the mixture from liquid herbal tinctures. In this case, one 5 cm teaspoonful should be taken three times a day after meals.

Children's eczema tonic

25 g (1 oz) fig wort
25 g (1 oz) dried nettles
25 g (1 oz) red clover

This tonic is suitable for small children over the age of one and may be sweetened with honey or maple syrup to make it more palatable. Any child suffering from severe eczema should be taken to see a qualified medical herbalist for specialist treatment.

Make up as an infusion, or a liquid tincture mixture as before (see page 98). Take three times daily after meals as above.

Internal psoriasis tonic

25 g (1 oz) mountain grape
25 g (1 oz) burdock root
25 g (1 oz) sasparilla
25 g (1 oz) yellow dock root
25 g (1 oz) red clover flowers

Psoriasis is another distressing disorder that is a distant relation of eczema and also responds well to internal treatment. A diet low in saturated animal fats but high in essential fatty acids is important. Daily supplements of evening primrose oil and cod liver oil are often helpful, together with beta carotene and zinc. Medical herbalists are often able to treat this distressing disorder and the following herbal tonic may also be useful, but be prepared for the condition to worsen before seeing an improvement. Sea water baths are also helpful (see the psoriasis salt water bath on page 126).

Mix together the dried ingredients and make an infusion by mixing 25 g (1 oz) of the herbal blend with 600 ml (1 pint) water. Drink 3 small cupfuls daily after breakfast, lunch and dinner.

The herbs may be bought dried from a herbal supplier and made up daily. Alternatively, a medical herbalist or herbal supplier can make up a mixture from liquid herbal tinctures. In this case, one 5 ml teaspoon should be taken three times a day after meals.

Instant beauty boosters

Rapid cleansers
- Use plain, live yoghurt to cleanse the skin and remove dirt and make-up. Simply rub into the skin and splash off with tepid water.
- Mix together 15 ml (1 tbsp) finely ground oatmeal with 30 ml (2 tbsp) hot water, gently rub into the skin and rinse off.
- Use jojoba oil or grapeseed oil to shift stubborn waterproof mascara. Apply with a lightly dampened cotton wool pad.

Simple skin tonics
- Warm chamomile tea is an excellent skin toner for dry, sensitive skins.
- Pure rosewater makes a refreshing skin tonic. Try using it straight from the fridge.
- To remove soap-sud residues and restore the skin's natural pH (acid/alkaline) balance, mix 5 ml (1 tsp) cider vinegar into a large tumbler of cool water and splash over the face after cleansing.

Spot busters
- dab on neat acetone to dry up stubborn spots using a fresh cotton-tipped applicator for each pimple.
- apply dots of milk of magnesia liquid to heal skin blemishes and acne lesions.
- use neat witch hazel on a cotton wool ball to clear a spotty forehead or chin.

Open-pore tonics
- Apply a small quantity of neat vodka to the nose and chin area to tighten enlarged pores.
- A slice of lemon rubbed over the affected area helps open pores appear smaller and also fades freckles.

Skin scrubbers

- 15 ml (1 tbsp) granulated white sugar mixed with a few drops of hot water makes an excellent skin scrub for slightly spotty skins, as sugar has mild anti-bacterial properties.
- Before stepping into the shower, smooth olive oil over the body and run in handfuls of finely ground sea salt for an invigorating all-over skin scrub.
- Massage a handful of coarsely ground oatmeal on the chest and upper arms while in the bath to leave the skin soft and glowing.

Speedy skin nourishers

- To re-moisturise a dry, sallow complexion, massage a generous dollop of fresh mayonnaise into the skin, leave for ten minutes and rinse with cool water.
- A thin layer of sunflower or soya margarine serves as a good make-shift moisturiser.
- A small amount of almond oil or avocado oil will nourish the face and neck. Apply before bedtime and leave overnight to sink into the skin.

6

Moisturisers and Skin Creams

Our skin makes its own moisturiser by mixing water with a
natural oil called sebum, which is secreted by the sebaceous
glands. Sebum is produced from these tiny glands that lie
just beneath the surface of the skin, and flows along ducts
into the hair follicles and on to the skin. Sebum itself is
slightly acidic and has an anti-bacterial action to protect the
skin from germs. The production of sebum is heavily in-
fluenced by our hormones, which is why skintypes vary so
much from person to person. Modern living also affects
sebum and the overall moisture levels in our skin.

Centrally heated environments and air-conditioned offices
rob the complexion of the moisture it needs to stay supple
and young looking. Extreme weather conditions such as the
wind, sun and low humidity levels also conspire against the
complexion and encourage dehydration. In addition, the
skin's ability to retain moisture reduces with age, which is
why our skin tends to become dryer as we get older. Other
factors that deplete our natural moisture levels within the

skin include smoking, alcohol and a diet low in essential fatty acids such as vegetable oils. Using a moisturising cream is a good way of topping up the skin's moisture content, not by adding more oil, but by forming a protective film over the surface of the skin that prevents valuable water from escaping.

There are two main types of moisturising creams for the face and body. Water-in-oil emulsions are the richest form of cream that suit dry, sensitive and more mature skintypes. These are especially useful during the winter months when the skin is more prone to flaking and chapping. The other type of cream is made with an oil-in-water formulation which means that it is lighter, more easily absorbed and suits normal, combination and oily skins (even oily complexions may need a light-weight moisturiser occasionally, as skin dehydration is caused by water evaporating from within the skin, not a lack of sebum on its surface). This type of lighter skin cream is more useful in the humid summer months as they generally contain humectants such as glycerine, which attract moisture from the atmosphere. They are not so good in dry air conditions as they tend to attract precious moisture from the skin itself.

These days, modern moisturisers have many added skin benefits. They may contain sunscreens that give the face anti-ageing protection from the sun's rays, an increasingly important consideration as the ozone layer thins above us. Skin creams may also contain soothing ingredients such as antiseptic herbal extracts to help heal irritations. They also help to shield the skin from atmospheric pollutants such as car fumes and cigarette smoke and comprise a very valuable barrier cream. The best time to use a moisturiser is immediately after cleansing the face. If your skin is very dry you can apply a thin layer of cream to the skin while it is still damp as this helps trap extra moisture. Night creams are also useful if your skin is dry or showing visible signs of ageing. The best type of night creams are made with just a few simple ingredients, such as rejuvenating and soothing herbal extracts which have plenty of time to penetrate the skin while we sleep.

Rich geranium moisturiser

60 ml (2¼ fl oz) avocado oil
60 ml (2¼ fl oz) wheatgerm oil
25 ml (1 fl oz) lanolin
5 ml (1 tsp) beeswax pieces
30 ml (2 tbsp) rosewater
2.5 ml (½ tsp) borax powder
10–15 drops geranium essential oil

This emollient cream makes a lovely night-time treatment or rich daily moisturiser and suits even sensitive skins.

Place the avocado and wheatgerm oils together in a ceramic basin and put inside a saucepan half-filled with water. Add the lanolin and beeswax pieces and heat gently until the mixture has completely melted.

Meanwhile, dissolve the borax powder in the rosewater and add to the waxy mixture. Stir thoroughly and remove from the heat. Continue to stir the mixture until it is cool enough to transfer into small screw-top jars.

Honey bee moisturiser

60 ml (2 fl oz) almond oil
60 ml (2 fl oz) avocado oil
60 g (2 oz) cocoa butter
20 g (2 tsp) runny honey
10 drops chamomile essential oil

This smooth skin cream smells delicious and is mildly anti-bacterial due to its honey content.

Place the almond oil, avocado oil, cocoa butter and beeswax pieces in a ceramic bowl and put inside a saucepan that has been half-filled with water. Heat gently over a low flame until the cocoa butter and beeswax have melted.

Remove from the heat and stir in the runny honey. Beat continuously with a metal spoon or palette knife. Continue to stir while the mixure cools, add the chamomile essential oil and pour into a small screw-top jar. Store in a cool, dark place.

This is a concentrated moisturiser so use sparingly and if you find that the honey starts to separate out simply stir it back into the mixture.

Chamomile neck cream

50 ml (2 fl oz) strong chamomile tea
10 g (½ oz) beeswax pieces
50 g (2 oz) cocoa butter
30 ml (2 tbsp) almond or avocado oil
2 drops chamomile essential oil

This rich throat cream is especially suitable for using on areas of severely dehydrated skin such as the upper arms and elbows.

Make the chamomile tea by infusing 1 dessertspoonful (10 ml) of dried chamomile flowers or 1 herb tea bag in a cupful of almost-boiling water. Allow to steep for several minutes before straining.

Meanwhile, melt the beeswax and cocoa butter in a small saucepan and stir in the almond or avocado oil (the avocado oil is more nourishing). Remove from the heat and pour in 30 ml (2 tbsp) of the chamomile tea, stir vigorously and add the 2 drops of essential oil. Continue to stir until the mixture is cool enough to be transferred into small jars. Seal each one with a small disc of greaseproof paper and a screw-top lid.

To use, scoop out a small amount and warm between the palms of the hands before smoothing on to the skin.

Oil-free moisturiser

20 g (¾ oz) linseeds
200 ml (7 fl oz) boiling water
15 ml (1 tbsp) glycerine
15 ml (1 tbsp) rosewater
1 drop neroli essential oil (optional)

Linseeds are an excellent source of natural mucilage, a gel-like paste that soothes the skin. To make, crack the linseeds open by whizzing in a blender or coffee grinder for a few seconds. Transfer them to a small cup and pour on the boiling water. Stir continually while the linseeds steep as the mixture cools down. Strain off the linseeds and discard.

Mix the linseed mucilage with the glycerine and rosewater to form a lightly moisturising lotion. Add the neroli essential oil to give the lotion the wonderful aroma of orange blossom.

Apply to combination or oily skins after cleansing.

Sensitive skin splash

120 ml (4 fl oz) rosewater
60 ml (2 fl oz) glycerine

This simple moisturising lotion is an excellent soother for sensitive skins. It also makes a wonderful after-bath body splash that leaves the skin smelling sweet and feeling smooth.

Whisk together the rosewater with the glycerine. Store in a tightly sealed bottle away from heat and light. Shake gently before use. Rosewater is available from most chemists or can be made by blending 25 ml (1 fl oz) essence of roses with 4.5 litres (8 pints) distilled water.

Cucumber shaving cream

175 g (6 oz) coconut oil
50 ml (2 fl oz) witch hazel
90 ml (6 tbsp) almond oil
15 ml (1 tbsp) cucumber juice
4 drops sandalwood essential oil
4 drops lavender essential oil

This subtly fragrant shaving cream is excellent for a man's bristly beard, or for softer hairs on feminine legs and under-arms. It contains cucumber juice to soothe the skin, lavender oil to heal any razor nicks and natural plant oils to leave the skin moisturised and smooth.

Melt the coconut oil slowly in a small saucepan over a low heat (coconut oil is solid at room temperature). Remove from the heat and stir in the witch hazel and almond oil. Make the cucumber juice by whizzing half a peeled cucumber in a blender and passing the liquid through a fine sieve.

Add the juice to the mixture together with the sandalwood and lavender essential oils. Mix thoroughly and pour into a screw-top jar.

To use, stir the cream with the fingertips and apply to the skin. After shaving, remove any remaining traces of cream with a hot damp flannel and pat the skin dry. There is no need to follow with an additional moisturiser as the skin will be left feeling smooth and comfortable.

Note: this formula contains fresh cucumber extracts which means it should be kept in a cool place and has a limited shelf-life.

Moisturising eye balm

10 ml (2 tsp) avocado oil
10 ml (2 tsp) wheatgerm oil
10 ml (2 tsp) calendula oil
2.5 ml (½ tsp) runny honey
10 g (2 tsp) cocoa butter

This mixture uses pure plant oils and honey to boost the moisture content of the fragile skin tissues surrounding the eye area. The honey is important because it is rich in natural sugars that are similar to the skin's own Natural Moisturising Factors (NMFs), which keep it nourished.

Place all the ingredients in a ceramic bowl and put into a larger saucepan that has been half-filled with water. Heat gently until the honey and cocoa butter have dissolved and dispersed into the plant oils.

Stir to ensure all the ingredients have mixed thoroughly together. Pour into a small bottle or screw-top jar and give the mixture a final stir to prevent it from separating out as it sets.

Apply at night, using light fingertip movements to pat around the entire eye area.

Luscious lip glosser

15 g (½ oz) beeswax pieces
25 g (1 oz) cocoa butter
35 ml (1 fl oz) castor oil
35 ml (1 fl oz) almond oil
8 drops clove essential oil

This lip balm moisturises, protects and shines the lips while also guarding against chapping and cold sores.

Place the beeswax pieces, cocoa butter, castor oil and almond oil into a ceramic bowl and put inside a saucepan that has been half-filled with water. Heat gently until the beeswax and cocoa butter have melted. Remove from the heat and allow to cool, stirring continually.

Add the drops of clove essential oil and pour into small tubs or jars. Tiny lip-gloss pots or clean make-up compacts make good containers. Alternatively, pour the mixture into small cylindrical moulds, such as plastic syringes available from the chemist. Place these in the fridge to cool and harden before transferring to an empty lipstick case.

Dew-drop body cream

120 ml (4 fl oz) almond oil
10 g (¼ oz) beeswax
50 g (2 oz) cocoa butter
350 ml (12 fl oz) herb tea (e.g., elderflower or rosehip)
8 drops lavender essential oil (optional)

This after-bath moisturiser encapsulates droplets of water that are absorbed by the skin as you rub it on. It is highly recommended as a regular treatment to keep the body sleek and smooth.

Place the almond oil, beeswax pieces and cocoa butter into a ceramic bowl and put inside a saucepan half-filled with water. Heat gently until the beeswax and cocoa butter have completely dissolved. Remove from the heat and add the water and lavender essential oil, stirring continuously whilst the mixture cools.

Pour into a tub or large screw-top jar. Keep beside the bath or shower and massage liberally into the body after bathing. Instead of using the lavender oil you can fragrance this mixture with any essential oil according to personal preference, such as rose, jasmine or neroli (orange blossom).

Facial suncream

50 g (2 oz) zinc oxide cream
25 ml (1 fl oz) castor oil
10 ml (2 tsp) arrowroot

Zinc oxide is an excellent sunblock as it contains particles that reflect the sun's harmful rays away from the face. This cream is also water-resistant and can be used if you are swimming in a pool or in the sea. As it does not contain chemical sun filters it is especially suitable for those with sensitive skins.

Mix together the zinc oxide cream and castor oil until they form a smooth paste. Add the arrowroot and stir thoroughly. Transfer to a small, screw-top jar and apply to clean skin before going out into the sun.

Sunscreen oil

120 ml (4 fl oz) sesame oil
50 ml (2 fl oz) grapeseed oil
50 ml (2 fl oz) strong tea (e.g., Darjeeling)

This is good sunscreening oil for skins that tan easily, and can be used all over the body. However, the sun-filtering properties are not good enough for those with fair skin, for children or for tropical climates.

Pour the oils together into a large, screw-top bottle, add the cooled tea and shake well. Sesame oil has natural sun-screening properties and will shield the skin from about one-third of the sun's harmful rays. The tannins present in the tea also help block ultra-violet light. Shake the mixture vigorously before applying.

7

The Anti-Agers

As medical science gradually unravels the mysteries of skin ageing, so the cosmetic chemists are constantly trying to catch up with creams, serums and lotions that will help to turn back the clock. The last decade has without doubt been the age of the 'wrinkle removers' and we have been bombarded with creams from the cosmetic counters that promise much and cost even more. There is little doubt that some of these so-called miracle creams are a complete waste of money, but the cosmetic scientists have turned up some interesting findings that we can all use in everyday skincare. For example, we now know that the sun is the skin's enemy number one. Unless we take steps to shield our faces from its glare our complexion quickly becomes wrinkly and slack almost as fast as a moisture-laden grape turns into a sun-dried raisin. Not only do the sun's rays destroy the supporting collagen and elastin fibres of the face but they also encourage deep brown pigmentation marks known as 'age' or liver spots. The very best anti-ageing cream of all is a total sunblock, such as a simple zinc oxide cream, that protects the complexion from the damage the sun does to the lower levels of the skin. Protection is always far easier than a cure and it is well worth taking steps in our early years to ensure that our face never shows the ravages of premature sun-induced skin ageing.

But for those of us who spent our earlier years outdoors, or who plainly refuse to give up sun-worshipping, there have been other skin-saving developments that can help keep the lines at bay. We now know that our skin responds to certain vitamins such as the anti-oxidants. This group of nutrients includes Vitamin C, Vitamin E and beta carotene (the vegetable form of Vitamin A). In recent years they have become increasingly newsworthy as medical researchers discovered that anti-oxidants can help many forms of chronic degenerative disease such as cancer, coronary heart disease, cataracts and even signs of skin ageing. Anti-oxidants work by protecting cells within the body from a kind of rusting process called oxidation. This occurs when cells come under attack from free radicals. Another modern medical buzz-word, free radicals are unstable particles that occur frequently within the body and cause a great deal of damage to our cells. Free radicals are on the increase because they are encouraged by factors of modern-day living such as chemical pollutants, smoking, stress and the increased ultra-violet light that is slipping through our depleted ozone layer.

In addition to the anti-oxidants there are several other types of nutrients that can ward off wrinkles. For example, the essential fatty acids are a group of important nutrients that help strengthen skin cells and keep them looking young. Found mainly in oily foods such as vegetable oils, avocados and oily fish, essential fatty acids are a valuable part of our diet as they act as internal moisturisers by strengthening skin cells from within. But the essential fatty acids and the anti-oxidant vitamins are not only important in our diet, they are also useful when applied directly to the surface of the skin. Vitamins A and E can penetrate the surface of the skin, and it has also been proven clinically that some essential fatty acids help severe skin disorders when applied topically, as sometimes happens when evening primrose oil is rubbed on to patches of eczema. Other scientific discoveries that help to slow down the formation of fine lines and wrinkles include the identification of certain fruit acids from plant extracts, the anti-oxidant properties of common herbs such as sage, parsley and thyme, and the powers of some essential oils to repair damaged skin.

Other important treatments to ward off wrinkles include exfoliation, exercise and massage. All three activities really do work because they boost the amount of blood brought to the surface of the skin, which carries with it fresh oxygen supplies. Oxygen is essential for healthy skin cell functioning and it is important to encourage sufficient supplies to reach the surface of the skin. Any form of exercise will benefit the complexion, even if it is only a brisk walk around the block. Massage also encourages increased blood flow to the skin's surface and is a wonderfully relaxing way of working out the face without moving a muscle.

Both exercise and massage also improve lymphatic drainage, which carries away toxins and cellular debris from beneath the surface of the skin. The lymphatic system runs parallel to the circulatory system throughout the body but, unlike the blood circulation, it does not have a heart to pump it around. Instead, the lymphatic system relies on regular movements in the form of daily exercise or massage to keep it flowing smoothly. There is no doubt that by encouraging our lymphatic system to work harder we can quickly improve skin tone and luminosity – and literally wipe *years* off our faces far faster than any skin cream ever invented. Exfoliation also supports lymphatic drainage to a lesser extent, but has the added benefit of stimulating skin cell renewal. By gently buffing off dead cells from the skin's surface we automatically speed up the rate at which fresh, plump skin cells are produced to replace them. This in turn leads to clearer, smoother-looking skin.

In recent years we have learnt a great deal about the ways in which our skin ages and exactly what action is needed to slow down the signs of visible ageing. Using a sunblock is vital during the summer months and may even become essential during the winter, too, if our ozone layer continues to be depleted at the current rate. Diet is also a key factor in our over-all health and has a profound impact on our skin's appearance. By increasing our intake of fresh, unprocessed foods, such as whole grains, olive oil, fruits and vegetables that are rich in essential fatty acids and the anti-oxidant nutrients we can expect our skin to retain its youthful glow. Adding a daily exercise session, massage or exfoliation treatment is also important to help preserve long-term good looks. But, in addition to these guidelines, there are a few highly specific treatments that we can make to give our skin cells a boost and supply them with the ingredients our complexion needs to remain supple, healthy and strong.

Nourishing cream

25g (1 oz) cocoa butter
25 g (1 oz) lanolin
25 g (1 fl oz) avocado oil
15 ml (1 tbsp) wheatgerm oil
4 evening primrose oil capsules
10 drops neroli essential oil
10 drops frankincense essential oil

A wonderfully rich moisturiser that contains all the nutrients the skin needs to repair itself whilst we sleep.

Put the cocoa butter and lanolin into a ceramic jug or bowl and place this inside a saucepan that has been half-filled with water. Heat on top of the stove until the mixture has completely melted. Stir in the avocado oil, wheatgerm oil and contents of the evening primrose oil capsules (pierce with a pin and squeeze out the oil).

Remove from the heat and stir continually while the mixture cools. When the mixture has cooled to around body temperature, add the drops of essential oils and pour into small screw-top jars. Use as a nourishing night cream for the face and neck.

Fast facial firmer

25 ml (1 fl oz) witch hazel
1 tsp cider vinegar
1 egg white

This facial firmer was first used by the Elizabethans, who actually left it on their faces all day to give the skin a smooth, glazed appearance. It is a useful treatment to brighten and tighten the complexion temporarily.

Mix together the witch hazel with the cider vinegar. Lightly beat the egg white until it starts to foam but not stiffen. Splash the mixture over freshly cleansed skin, smooth on the foaming egg whites and leave on the face and neck for 15 minutes, before rinsing off with cool water.

Skin smoother

25 g (1 oz) brewer's yeast powder
60 ml (4 tbsp) fresh apple juice
30 ml (2 tbsp) plain, live yoghurt

This treatment is especially suited to mature, greying complexions in need of a boost. Brewer's yeast is our best natural source of the B-complex vitamins and is also rich in RNA (ribonucleic acid) and DNA (deoxyribonucleic acid), the basis of all living cells. Before each skin cell dies, DNA issues an order to RNA to reproduce itself. Therefore, our skin cells should reproduce themselves exactly as before. However, as our RNA and DNA break down over time the reproduction process also degenerates. Some studies show that external application of RNA and DNA, as in the form of brewer's yeast, may help skin cells rejuvenate themselves.

Dissolve the brewer's yeast powder in the apple juice (freshly pressed is best as it still retains useful levels of enzymes). Stir in the plain, live yoghurt to form a smooth paste.

Apply to freshly cleansed skin on the face and neck, leave for 15 minutes and rinse off thoroughly with plenty of tepid water. Follow with a layer of rich moisturiser.

Tired eye tonic

25 ml (1 fl oz) chamomile tea
25 ml (1 fl oz) witch hazel
5 ml (1 tsp) castor oil
2 drops frankincense essential oil

The perfect treatment for puffy eyes, it leaves the delicate tissues around the eye area feeling refreshed and smooth.

Make the chamomile tea by infusing 1 dessertspoonful (10 ml) of dried chamomile flowers or 1 herb tea bag with a cup of almost-boiling water. Allow to cool. Mix together the witch hazel and place in a screw-top jam jar. Add the castor oil and 2 drops of frankincense essential oil.

Shake vigorously to combine the water-based extracts with the castor oil. Dip several cotton wool pads into the tonic, squeeze to remove excess liquid and place over the eye area. Alternatively, apply to skin using a piece of muslin cloth or clean face flannel. Leave in place for 10–15 minutes before removing. Store the remaining tonic in the fridge (using chilled tonic straight from the fridge is especially refreshing if eyes are sore or puffy).

Fast-acting massage oil

25 ml (1 fl oz) jojoba oil
25 ml (1 fl oz) wheatgerm oil
5 evening primrose oil capsules
3 drops frankincense essential oil

This nourishing facial oil is an excellent treatment for tired, devitalised and more mature skins. It is rich in essential fatty acids and the anti-ageing Vitamin E. It also contains frankincense essential oil, which is traditionally used in aromatherapy to rejuvenate the skin and leave the complexion with a youthful bloom.

Blend the jojoba and wheatgerm oils together in a bowl or jar. Pierce the evening primrose oil capsules with a pin and squeeze out their contents into the mixture. Add the 3 drops of frankincense essential oil.

Stir or shake well to ensure all the oils have mixed together thoroughly. Using the tips of the fingers only, massage into freshly cleansed skin on the face and neck. Use small circular movements to stimulate blood flow and lymphatic drainage beneath the surface of the skin. This is an ideal treatment to use just before going to bed as the oils are so rich they may feel slightly sticky on the skin. Leaving them on the face overnight gives the blend time to penetrate more deeply into the skin and means you will wake up with a softer, smoother complexion.

Moisture booster

½ small ripe avocado
1 egg yolk
5 ml (1 tsp) olive oil

This simple recipe gives the skin an instant 'fix' of moisture and is one of the fastest to make.

Mix together the ripe avocado, egg yolk and olive oil until the ingredients combine to form a smooth paste. Apply to clean skin on the throat, neck and upper chest area (you may find it easier to use a large make-up brush or pastry brush to paint the face mask on to the skin). Relax for 15–20 minutes to give the emollient ingredients sufficient time to penetrate the upper levels of the skin. Remove with tissues or dampened cotton wool pads.

Avocado revitaliser

½ small ripe avocado with skin and stone
15 ml (1 tbsp) plain, live yoghurt
5 ml (1 tsp) runny honey
5 ml (1 tsp) fresh lemon juice

Remove the skin from the halved avocado and set to one side. Mix the avocado together with the live yoghurt, runny honey and lemon juice until the mixture forms a smooth paste. Take the avocado skin and gently rub the inside part of the skin over the face and neck. This helps dislodge dead skin cells and prepares the skin for the revitalising face pack. Next, smooth the avocado mixture on to the face and throat, and relax for 10–15 minutes. Before rinsing away with warm water, gently rub the avocado stone over the face and neck. The action of rubbing the avocado stone stimulates pressure points on the face and boosts lymphatic drainage. It also increases blood circulation and gives the complexion an invigorating work-out.

Fine skin refiner

25 g (1 oz) ground almonds
15 ml (1 tbsp) runny honey
1 egg white

This is a two-in-one treatment that especially suits dry, fragile skins. The almonds are rich in natural oils and the essential fatty acids that feed the skin. They are best when freshly ground in a coffee grinder, as this ensures that they are not stale and rancid. When applied to the skin, the almonds and honey re-moisturise, while the egg white tightens upper tissues. Before rinsing away, the mixture can be used as a very gentle skin scrub to leave the face, neck and décolletage glowing.

Mix together the finely ground almonds with the runny honey until they form a thick, sticky paste. Lightly beat the egg white so that it is still liquid but has doubled in volume. Stir into the almond and honey paste.

Apply to clean skin on the throat, neck, shoulders and upper chest area. Relax for 15–20 minutes. Before washing away with warm water, lightly massage the mixture into the skin using light circular movements with the fingertips. Rinse the skin thoroughly before applying a light moisturiser.

Linseed tissue toner

30 ml (2 level tbsp) linseeds
60 ml (4 tbsp) hot water
2 drops cypress essential oil (optional)
piece of muslin cloth or cotton gauze

This treatment uses a warm linseed poultice to draw out excess fluid from puffy skin and firm up slackened skin tissues. Linseeds are rich in mucilages, which gently tighten and tone the skin, leaving it soft and sooth. The cypress essential oil is optional, but is especially useful to add if you have broken veins. This is because it acts as a vaso-dilator and as such helps shrink broken blood capillaries, reducing their appearance.

First, put the linseeds in a grinder and whizz for a few seconds, just to split open the seeds. Mix these with sufficient hot water to form a thick, gel-like paste. Add the cypress essential oil (if using) and stir thoroughly.

Spread the mixture on to half the piece of muslin cloth or cotton gauze, folding the other half over to seal the poultice. Place over the lower half of the face and neck and leave for 10 minutes. To speed up the process, place a small towel over the top which will seal in the heat.

Hot linseed compresses also work well on specific areas of the face and body that need toning up. For example, a twice-weekly treatment on the chin and neck is an excellent way to help firm a double chin. Larger poultices can also be made and applied to areas of cellulite on the stomach, hips and thighs. These may be covered with clingfilm to intensify the process. Regular use, i.e., twice a week for at least a month, is important for best results.

8

Baths and Body Care

The body is covered in an extremely large expanse of skin and yet, compared to our faces, it receives very little attention. Although the skin on the body spends most of its time under wraps, it has the same requirements for cleansing and moisturising as the face and neck. In fact, the body often needs more specialised care to treat specific problems such as severe dehydration, skin flaking, cellulite, water retention and areas of hardened, chapped skin. Fortunately, the treatments for such problems are often quick and simple, and most rely on natural plant and herbal ingredients for their active extracts. The only other equipment you need is a bath and/or shower to turn your home into a natural beauty salon.

HERBAL BATHS

The art of using herbal baths to treat skin and circulatory disorders is known as hydrotherapy. It is widely used on the

Continent and many European health spas offer several
types of healing baths to produce different effects within the
body. These 'water cures' often involve special mineral
waters or salt water from the sea. They may also be combined
with mud or seaweed body treatments to boost the metabolism and stimulate the skin. There are an infinite number
of possibilities when creating herbal baths, depending upon
the herb extracts used and the temperature and volume of
the water.

The best way to add herbal and plant extracts to bath water
is to sew them inside a small muslin bag which can be dan-
gled from the tap so the water releases a fresh infusion as it
flows through it. A small cotton drawstring bag is also useful
as it can be washed and re-used many times. Alternatively,
herb tea bags make a wonderfully simple addition to any
bath and there are now several hundred varieties to choose
from. Jacuzzis or whirlpool baths are also popular in health
spas and beauty salons and are good to stimulate blood
circulation and ease muscular stiffness.

However, do not sit in a hot tub for more than ten minutes
as it can make you feel faint and dizzy, and those with low
blood pressure or heart problems should avoid them alto-
gether. At home, even something as basic as the temperature
of the bath water is important. Warm baths are the most
soothing as they help relax tense muscles and calm fragile
nerves. These are also the best type to take after exercise as
they help prevent stiffness in the joints and muscles. Thera-
peutically, warm baths are used to treat mild colds, urinary
problems and low fevers. Both hot baths of temperatures of
100°F or more and cold baths are essentially shock treatments
for the body. Hot baths cause the pulse to increase and may
leave you feeling weak and drained. Prolonged hot baths put
the heart under unnecessary strain as the blood vessels ex-
pand in an attempt to cool the body. However, they can be
useful to induce sweating and therefore good for eliminating
toxins from the system. Cold baths also increase the rate at
which the heart beats, although the pulse slows down once it
has recovered from the initial shock. Cold baths can be especially helpful for boosting the blood circulation and toning
the skin.

Few things are as relaxing as wallowing in a full bath and
these are also the best for skin treatments as the entire body

is submerged. Half-filled baths tend to be cooler and are less of a strain on the system, so better for those with low blood pressure. The sitz-bath (see page 125) is an Austrian invention and involves sitting in just a few inches of water. Many European health spas have specially designed sitz-baths, but you can use an ordinary bath and hang your legs over the side so that just your waist, bottom and upper thighs are covered by the water. Believe it or not, the best sitz-baths are taken cold – and once the body has recovered from the initial jolt it is amazing how quickly the condition of the skin improves. Although I am not especially brave, I try and take a quick cold dip at least two or three times a week as it really does get the blood circulation going.

The most minimal form of hydrotherapy is the footbath, which not only benefits the feet but can also invigorate the rest of the body depending on which herbal extracts are added to it. Over all, hydrotherapy has to be one of the easiest and most under-rated forms of health and beauty treatments, and it is well worth experimenting with some of the following variations.

Relaxing baths

- To encourage a peaceful night, fill a muslin bag with a dried herbal mixture designed to induce sleep and hang it under the hot tap. The herbs with most powerful sedative effects are valerian, lemon balm, marjoram, lavender, hops and passion flower. Alternatively, make a similar brew using herb tea bags and add to warm bath water.

- Add cold chamomile tea or two chamomile tea bags to a warm bath to help relax the muscles and delicately scent the skin.
- The following herbal mixture is useful for soothing strained muscles and relieving tension in the joints: Infuse 5 ml (1 tsp) each of dried sage leaves, lavender flowers and chopped bay leaves in 1 cup of almost boiling water. Leave for 20 minutes. Strain then add the liquid to a pre-run warm bath.
- A few drops of essential oil transform an ordinary bath into a hedonistic indulgence. The most relaxing essences are lavender, lemon balm (melissa), sandalwood and bergamot. Always add the oils to a pre-run bath as they are broken down by heat and quickly loose their potency.

Invigorating baths

- To stimulate the circulation and aid the digestion add a rosemary herbal infusion to the bath. Place 50 g (2 oz) fresh rosemary leaves and stalks in 600 ml (1 pint) of boiling water and leave to infuse for 15 minutes before pouring into the bath water.
- Adding peppermint to a cool bath is a traditional way of pepping up the body. Place dried peppermint inside a muslin sachet before adding to the bath water or simply add a handful of freshly chopped leaves and flowering tops. Leftover peppermint tea can also be saved and added to the bath.
- The most invigorating essential oils are the citrus oils such as lemon and mandarin, as well as rosemary, jasmine and peppermint (do not add more than a couple of drops of peppermint as its high menthol content can make the skin feel cold).

Moisturising baths

- Take a tip from Cleopatra and her ass's milk by adding 15 ml (1 tbsp) dried milk powder to a pre-run warm bath to soften the skin while you soak.
- Make cotton sachets filled with finely ground oatmeal and place in the bath while the water is running. Once in the

bath, use the sachet to gently scrub away dead, dingy skin cells from the upper arms, hips and thighs.

- Add 10 ml (2 tsp) olive oil or sunflower oil to the bath water just before stepping in. This leaves the skin feeling so soft that you won't need to use a body lotion afterwards.
- Keep a jar of coconut oil in the bathroom and add a spoonful to each bath. For a more exotic skin treat, stir a few drops of rose or jasmine essential oil into the coconut oil. Just 3–4 drops is enough to subtly scent a small jar of coconut oil and the scent will last for ages.

HEALING BATHS

Fast footbaths

The footbath is a simple, straightforward treatment that can help a wide range of ailments. Ideally, the water should completely cover the feet and come halfway up the calves. Cold footbaths are good for reviving tired feet, and naturopaths often recommend them to ease headaches and insomnia. The feet should be submerged in the cold water for as long as possible or until the feet start to feel warm. Alternating between hot and cold footbaths is a time-honoured way to boost the blood circulation and can help prevent varicose veins in the legs. Feet and calves should first be placed in the hot footbath for two minutes, then plunged into cold water for one minute. This routine should be repeated ten times for maximum benefit.

Adding a few drops of lemon and peppermint essential oils to each footbath also helps to boost the blood flow and leaves the feet smelling fresh. Mustard footbaths are also a good way to ward off chilblains and help coughs and colds. Simply add 10 ml (2 tsp) strong English mustard to a hot footbath before soaking the feet for 15–20 minutes. Alternatively, add 15 ml (2 tsp) freshly grated ginger root to help ward off influenza.

The sitz-bath

As mentioned briefly at the beginning of the chapter, a cold sitz-bath is the most effective method of getting the circu-

lation going. It is also specifically good for reducing haemorrhoids (piles) and for improving the appearance of varicose
veins and small thread veins in the legs. Carried out
regularly, a cold sitz-bath reduces signs of cellulite, improves
the texture of the skin on buttocks and thighs and helps with
weight loss by stimulating the metabolism. It is a wonderful
treatment for those who sit still for most of the day as it prevents the blood from pooling in the lower half of the body. It
is also a great way to revive the body after a stressful day's
work.

A cold sitz-bath is quick, easy and not particularly painful:
Half fill the bath with cold water (during the winter months a
small amount of hot water may be added to ensure the water
is not icy, but it is important that the water is cold – not luke-
warm). Sit down in the bath bottom first, leaving your legs
dangling over the side. The water should cover you from
waist to upper thigh only. It makes the process far more plea-
sant if you leave your socks on to keep the feet warm and you
can also wrap a towel or cardigan around the upper half of
the body. Remain in the water for two minutes before getting
out and briskly rubbing the skin dry. The sitz-bath takes
almost no time at all and can be carried out every day if
desired. To see the maximum benefits it should be used at
least three times a week.

BATHS FOR SKIN PROBLEMS

Eczema

To help soothe the itch and irritation of eczema, psoriasis and
dermatitis, make an oat bran decoction to add to the bath
water. In a saucepan place 30 ml (2 tbsp) wheat bran with 30
ml (2 tbsp) oatmeal or porridge oat flakes and 600 ml (1 pint)
water and gently bring to the boil. Remove from the heat and
pass through a sieve. Add the milky liquid to a warm – not
hot – bath, just before stepping in.

Psoriasis

Inflamed and itchy skin conditions can be relieved by adding
sea water minerals to the bath water. The best come from the
Dead Sea in Israel, where people with skin disorders go

specifically to swim in its mineral-dense waters. Some healthfood shops sell packets of sea water minerals from the Dead Sea to add to the bath, otherwise use two or three handfuls of sea salt combined with a few strips of dried culinary seaweed or 15ml (1 tbsp) kelp powder to re-create the effect.

Itchy skin

Dry, sensitive skin is often caused when the skin's natural, acidic pH balance is disrupted. Avoid using soap in the bath (try the *Soapwort cleanser* on page 82) and add 15 ml (1 tbsp) of cider vinegar to restore the correct acid/alkaline ratio. It is also worth adding a splash of aloe vera juice to help calm skin irritations.

Sunburn

The most important factor when treating sunburn is to cool the skin down quickly, to prevent the heat from penetrating the lower levels of the skin. Soaking in a deep, cool bath rapidly brings down body temperature, and adding a handful of oatmeal or porridge oats also helps soothe angry, inflamed tissues. A few drops of lavender essential oil is also a wonderful skin soother, and a natural antiseptic that works especially well on sunburned skin. Vitamin E in the form of wheatgerm oil or from Vitamin E capsules is also a useful addition to re-moisturise the skin and helps prevent peeling while reducing the risk of blisters.

Bathtime skin treatments

Dry skin brushing is one of the best all-round beauty treatments, and it can be carried out just before stepping into the bath or shower. It is a terrific treatment for dingy skin, cellulite and for improving a sluggish circulation. The best time to do dry skin brushing is first thing in the morning, just before bathing. You will need a natural-fibre body brush or massage mitt that feels firm, but not too harsh, on the skin. Starting with the soles of the feet, brush the legs from feet to thighs using strong, sweeping movements. Concentrate on the lymphatic drainage points located at the backs of the knees and towards the groin, to increase the flow of lymph and assist the removal of toxins from the system. Pay particular attention to the backs of the thighs and buttocks to help break down fatty deposits from beneath the surface of the skin and reduce the appearance of cellulite. Carry on up the body, working gently over the stomach, sides and chest (avoiding the nipples). Brush up each arm, starting from the wrist and finishing on the upper inside arm.

Always brush towards the heart, as this is the way the lymph flows, and rinse the brush thoroughly after use. Dry skin brushing may feel strange and uncomfortable at first but it is well worth the effort. It increases the metabolism, improves skin tone, dislodges dingy skin cells and literally gets the whole body skin glowing (if you stand against the light while you brush you will see hundreds of dead skin cells flying off the body).

BODY SCRUBS

Other methods for improving the skin's texture and tone include body scrubs. These are best carried out either before or during a shower, as they tend to be quite a messy treatment. Body scrubs involve massaging the skin with a gritty substance to shift dead skin cells and embedded grime, and improve the appearance of spots and pimples. They can be used either on their own or in conjunction with a rough flannel or loofah to increase their effectiveness. Loofahs themselves are the long, fibrous pod of the *Luffa aegyptiaca* plant, which has been used as a body scrubber since Ancient Egyptian times. Massage pads and mitts can be made from pieces of loofah and these are good for scrubbing smaller areas of skin such as the hands and the soles of the feet. Loofahs should be kept clean by rinsing in clean water after each use and should be hung to dry to prevent them from becoming mouldy.

Basic body scrub

100 g (4 oz) granulated white sugar
100 g (4 oz) finely ground sea salt
100 g (4 oz) coarsely ground oatmeal

This simple mixture is made from ingredients found on most kitchen shelves, yet is just as effective as expensive skin exfoliators.

Mix the ingredients together in a large bowl and transfer to a screw-top jar. To use, pour a small amount into the palm of the hand and massage into dampened skin. Rinse thoroughly. These three ingredients work well together as the sugar is mildly anti-bacterial and helps heal minor skin irritations, the salt is an efficient body buffer, while the oatmeal soothes the skin as it gently dislodges dead skin cells. Keep the jar in the bathroom as the mixture is gentle enough to use each time you take a shower.

Peanut butter scrub

50 g (2 oz) crunchy peanut butter
25 g (1 oz) finely ground sea salt
30 ml (2 tbsp) almond oil

This body scrub tastes good enough to eat! It is also rich in natural oils that leave the skin feeling soft and smooth.

Mix together the peanut butter with the sea salt and stir in the almond oil. The mixture should form a soft paste. Rub on to damp skin, all over the body, concentrating on areas of hard skin on the elbows, upper arms and knees. Rinse off with warm water and shower as usual.

Bust scrub

25 g (1 oz) medium ground oatmeal
25 g (1 oz) finely ground almonds
15 ml (1 tbsp) almond oil

Most skin scrubs are too abrasive to use on the delicate skin that covers the breasts, but a gentle skin scrub is a good way to preserve skin tone and to remove any flakiness from the breasts or nipple area.

Mix together the oatmeal and the almonds with the almond oil to form a paste. Apply to dampened skin and massage into the neck and chest area with firm but gentle circular movements. Always massage upwards to avoid pulling the skin and encouraging slackening.

Rinse thoroughly and shower as usual. You will find the skin is left feeling especially soft and smooth.

Hip and thigh scrub

30 ml (2 tbsp) grapeseed oil
5 drops juniper essential oil
2 drops lemon essential oil
75 g (3 oz) polenta or cornmeal

This is my favourite body treatment as it is very simple to do and really works wonders on the skin. It is ideal for shifting patches of stubborn cellulite and should be carried out at least twice a week to see the best results.

In a screw-top bottle or jar, mix together the grapeseed oils with the essential oils and shake well. Pour the oil mixture over the cornmeal and mix to form a gritty paste. Apply to dampened skin on the hips, buttocks and thighs. Massage firmly, using sweeping, circular movements in an upwards direction.

For greater effect, use a rough flannel or massage mitt instead of the hands. Massage for at least 2 minutes before rinsing the gritty particles away. Any mixture left over can be rubbed into the feet, hands and upper arms to leave them exceptionally smooth and glowing.

MUD PACKS

Probably the messiest beauty treatment of all is the mud pack. Often used on the face and neck, it takes a real natural beauty enthusiast to try an all-over body pack, but the results are worth the extra effort. Mud packs work by using a mixture of natural clays to draw out embedded impurities, sebum and general grime from the pores of the skin. These clays also remove the top layer of dead skin cells, leaving the entire surface of the body soft, fresh and glowing. Mud packs may also be used for more localised treatments, such as areas of acne on the back, or cellulite on the hips and thighs.

Whole-body mud pack

150 g (5 oz) Fuller's earth
200 ml (7 fl oz) fresh apple juice
15 ml (1 tbsp) lemon juice
30 ml (2 tbsp) almond oil
15 ml (1 tbsp) runny honey
6 drops sandalwood or neroli essential oil

This all-over body treat is ideal to do just before a holiday, when you want your skin to look its best, or as an annual 'spring clean' to invigorate grey, dingy skin after the winter. It is extremely effective and costs a fraction of the price of expensive beauty salon body treatments.

Mix together the Fuller's earth with the apple juice and lemon juice until it forms a smooth paste. Stir in the almond oil, honey and fragrant essential oil. To use, apply small amounts of the mixture to the body, starting at the feet and working upwards. Concentrate on areas of dull, dingy skin such as the hips, thighs and upper arms.

Gently massage the mixture into the skin and leave for a few minutes to dry before stepping into the shower. Use warm water thoroughly to rinse away all traces of the mask, then shower as usual.

Anti-acne back pack

100 g (4 oz) Fuller's earth
2 egg whites, lightly beaten
5 ml (1 tsp) alum crystals
5 ml (1 tsp) sulphur powder
6 drops tea tree essential oil

You will need a partner or close friend to help apply this properly, as most acne spots occur in hard to reach places in the middle of the back.

Mix together the Fuller's earth and lightly beaten egg whites until they form a smooth paste (add a few drops of hot water if the mixture becomes too stiff to handle). Add the alum crystals, sulphur powder and tea tree essential oil. Stir well to combine all the ingredients.

Ask a friend or partner to massage the mixture into the back. Any leftover mixture may be used on the feet to smooth and soften hard skin. Leave the pack to dry out completely (approximately 15 minutes) before rinsing away with tepid water in the shower and gently patting the skin dry.

Anti-pimple mud-pack

50 g (2 oz) Fuller's earth
175 ml (6 fl oz) strong sage tea

This simple pack can be used on a spotty back or chest and is good for drawing toxins out of the skin.

First, make the sage tea by infusing 1 dessertspoonful (10 ml) dried sage in 1 cup almost-boiling water. Leave to steep for 10 minutes before using. Alternatively, add 4 drops sage essential oil to 1 cup of hot water.

Mix the sage tea together with the Fuller's earth to form a smooth paste. Apply to a freshly cleansed area of skin and leave to dry (approximately 10 minutes). Rinse away thoroughly, using cool, clean water and pat the skin dry.

THE MAGIC OF MASSAGE

The best way to follow any type of body treatment is with a gentle massage. The art of massage is the ultimate cure for stress, nervous tension and for promoting a feeling of overall well-being. In an ideal world we would all be massaged by our partners, but more often than not we must rely on various techniques of self-massage. However, these can be extremely effective in boosting blood circulation, stimulating lymphatic drainage, reducing the signs of cellulite and improving skin tone. The following are the most effective forms of self-massage:

- *Effleurage*. The basic stroking movements of Swedish massage, varying from light to firm pressure. Good as an initial treatment to warm and relax the muscles.
- *Do-In*. The traditional Oriental form of self-massage, based on tapping the body from top to toe. Designed to get the circulation going, and an excellent way to start the day.
- *Lymphatic Drainage*. This uses long sweeping movements, with the palms of the hands, that follow the lymphatic channels in the body in a direction towards the lymph nodes. The idea is to help drain away the toxins and impurities that collect in the lymphatic system. Lymph nodes are situated behind the knees, in the groin, under the arms and by the collarbones. Lymphatic drainage is a useful technique for anyone with fluid retention, cellulite or skin disorders.
- *Petrissage*. Another Swedish massage technique that uses kneading movements to reach the deeper levels of the skin, petrissage works on muscles, ligaments and the connective tissue to release areas of tension. The technique is similar to kneading bread dough and works well on fleshier areas of the body such as hips, stomach and thighs.
- *Tapotement*. This tapping movement is made by cupping the hands and gently slapping the body to produce a clapping sound. It is a quick, invigorating method of bringing fresh blood supplies to the surface of the skin.
- *Reflexology*. Mainly used on the feet where there are several hundred 'reflex zones'. These are nerve endings that correspond to areas and organs of the body. The theory is that

timulating these zones you automatically stimulate the
~rent parts of the body. Reflexology massage is easy to
ɔn your own feet by using the tips of the thumbs to
press lightly over the toes and sole of each foot. Other
areas of reflex zones include the hands and the ears and
these can be massaged in the same way.

- *Vibration*. The cheat's version of self-massage is to use an
  electronic vibrating gadget. Several designs are available,
  such as the G-5 machine used by professional beauty thera-
  pists to give a firm, deep massage that penetrates into the
  deepest muscle groups in the body. Home versions include
  hand-held anti-cellulite massagers designed to tone the
  skin by stimulating the blood supply and encouraging the
  breakdown of fatty deposits beneath the surface.

Massage oils

Whatever type of massage you choose, you will need to use a
massage oil. There are two main reasons for using an oil
while you massage. Firstly, an oil helps the hands glide
smoothly over the surface of the skin and reduces friction.
Secondly, the oil itself can be formulated to have moisturising and therapeutic properties which also benefit the body.

Basic body oil

100 ml (4 fl oz) grapeseed oil
5 ml (1 tsp) wheatgerm oil
10 drops lavender or sandalwood essential oil

An excellent everyday oil that will moisturise the skin after
bathing, grapeseed oil has the lightest texture and if used
sparingly, won't leave sticky traces on clothes. It is a good
idea to add a small amount of wheatgerm oil to each oil blend
as it has a high Vitamin E content and this nutrient is a
natural anti-oxidant and therefore prevents spoilage by
rancidity.

Mix the oils together and store in a screw-top bottle or jar.
Shake before use.

Athletic muscle rub

100 ml (4 fl oz) grapeseed oil
5 ml (1 tsp) wheatgerm oil
10 drops rosemary essential oil
5 drops lavender essential oil

This invigorating lotion is excellent for reviving a flagging physique and smells macho enough for the fussiest male!

Mix the oils together in a screw-top bottle and jar. Shake well before use and apply liberally to areas of the body where the muscles have been working hardest, e.g., the calves, thighs and biceps.

Re-moisturising body oil

50 ml (2 fl oz) avocado oil
50 ml (2 fl oz) almond oil
10 ml (2 tsp) wheatgerm oil
5 drops chamomile essential oil
5 drops sandalwood or geranium essential oil

This oil can be used for massage, and a splash may also be added to the bath if the skin is very dry. Especially good for areas of hardened, chapped skin on the hands, elbows and feet, as the avocado oil penetrates the surface layer of skin to moisturise below.

Mix all the oils together in a screw-top bottle or jar and shake well before use.

Anti-cellulite oil

100 ml (4 fl oz) grapeseed oil
5 ml (1 tsp) wheatgerm oil
10 drops juniper essential oil
5 drops lemon essential oil
5 drops fennel essential oil

This anti-cellulite formula is highly effective at breaking down the fatty deposits that lead to the dimpled, orange-peel effect on the thighs.

Mix all the oils together in a screw-top bottle or jar and shake well before use. Use daily on the hips and buttocks after bathing, massaging into the skin, using firm, circular movements.

Body lotions

Body oils are good for massage but there are times when we may want to use a body lotion that sinks in more quickly and leaves a trace of delicate perfume on the skin. The following recipes are especially good for dry skins that need regular moisturising to encourage a silky smooth feel.

Extra-rich body lotion

50 g (2 oz) cocoa butter
30 ml (2 tbsp) calendula oil
15 ml (1 tbsp) avocado oil
5 ml (1 tsp) wheatgerm oil
10 drops chamomile, neroli or sandalwood essential oil

This richly emollient skin lotion is excellent for the legs which have few sebaceous glands to keep them naturally moisturised. It is also good as an intensive hand cream or for smoothing chapped skin on the elbows and knees.

Place the cocoa butter in a small saucepan and melt gently over a low heat. Remove from the stove and stir in the calendula, avocado and wheatgerm oils. Allow the mixture to cool before adding the chamomile essential oil.

Pour into a large screw-top jar and apply liberally after bathing to dehydrated skin.

Rose petal body cream

15 g (½ oz) anhydrous lanolin
15 g (½ oz) cocoa butter
20 ml (4 tsp) almond oil
20 ml (4 tsp) glycerine (preferably vegetable)
6 drops rose essential oil

This richly moisturising cream smells delicious and is a wonderful treatment for areas of dry, chapped skin.

Place the lanolin and cocoa butter in a ceramic bowl and put this inside a saucepan that has been half-filled with water. Gently heat over a low flame until the beeswax has melted and the mixture forms a smooth paste. Remove from the heat and stir in the almond oil and glycerine (use vegetable glycerine if you prefer a cruelty-free cream).

Allow to cool before adding the rose essential oil, stirring well to distribute the fragrance (rosewood or rose geranium essential oils are good fragrance alternatives to the more expensive pure rose oil). Pour the mixture into a small jar and apply liberally to dry skin after bathing.

After-sun skin soother

25 ml (1 oz) cocoa butter
30 ml (2 tbsp) almond oil
15 ml (1 tbsp) olive oil
5 ml (1 tsp) wheatgerm oil
10 drops lavender essential oil

This semi-solid lotion is excellent for treating mild sunburn, preventing peeling and for prolonging a suntan. It is also deeply re-moisturising and may be used as an intensive skin conditioner on areas of parched skin.

Melt the cocoa butter in a small saucepan over a low heat. Add the almond, olive and wheatgerm oils and stir vigorously to mix. Allow to cool and add the lavender essential oil.

Pour the mixture into a screw-top bottle or jar.

9

Hand and Foot Care

Hands and feet are our hard-working extremities, and deserve pampering with a little extra care and attention. The skin that covers our hands and feet is much thicker than elsewhere on the body. This provides them with important protection during their arduous daily tasks, but can some-times result in a build-up of rough, chapped skin that looks unsightly and is often painful. Our hands especially are always out on constant show and are continually exposed to the elements. Strong sunshine encourages brown 'age' spots on the backs of the hands, cold weather leaves them dry and chapped, while washing in soapy water strips away their natural oils, leaving them rough and wrinkled.

Our feet come under a different kind of pressure as they carry our weight around all day, often squeezed into tightly fitting boots and shoes. During the winter months the skin on our feet may go for months without being allowed to breathe properly, as feet are cocooned in constant layers of thick tights, woolly socks and warm bedclothes. It is said that the expression on your face is due to the comfort of your feet and it is certainly true that corns, chilblains and bunions cause a great deal of misery. So it is hardly surprising that pedicures have become one of the most popular beauty treatments – a small amount of time spent looking after the feet can put a smile on the face all year round.

Fingernails and toenails also require regular care to keep them trim and attractive. Giving yourself a weekly manicure is a simple beauty treatment that keeps nails tidy and prevents problems such as splitting, flaking and painful in-growing toenails. The following remedies are easy to make and are well worth including in your regular beauty routine. Not only do they make the hands and feet look more attractive, but they also help prevent more serious disorders from developing in the future.

Cuticle cream

10 g (¼ oz) beeswax pieces
60 ml (4 tbsp) almond oil
5 drops lavender essential oil
10 drops tea tree essential oil

This nourishing cream also contains essential oils to heal minor skin irritations and help prevent fungal nail infections.

Place the beeswax pieces and almond oil together in a ceramic bowl and put inside a saucepan that has been half-filled with water. Heat gently on top of the stove until the beeswax has completely melted into the oil. Stir thoroughly, remove from the heat and allow to cool slightly. Add the essential oils and stir again.

Pour the mixture into a small screw-top jar and use to massage daily around the nails to soften cuticles and prevent them from splitting and peeling.

Lavender barrier cream

10 g (¼ oz) beeswax pieces
25 g (1 oz) cocoa butter
60 ml (4 tbsp) almond oil
15 ml (1 tbsp) castor oil
15 drops lavender essential oil

This waterproof hand cream will protect the hands from environmental abuse and is perfect to use before chores such as gardening and washing-up. Keep a tub handy in the kitchen for regular use. Instead of using lavender essential oil, the cream may also be scented with lemon or sandalwood oils for a more macho aroma.

Place the beeswax pieces and cocoa butter in a ceramic bowl and put this in a saucepan that has been half-filled with water. Heat gently on top of the stove until the beeswax and cocoa butter have melted together. Remove from the heat and stir in the almond oil and castor oil. Allow to cool and beat in the lavender essential oil.

Pour the mixture into tubs or shallow screw-top jars and rub into the hands whenever a protective barrier cream is needed.

Orange blossom massage cream

20 ml (1 fl oz) almond oil
40 ml (2 fl oz) olive or avocado oil
10 g (½ oz) beeswax pieces
20 ml (1 fl oz) rosewater
5 ml (1 tsp) lecithin granules, or 4 lecithin capsules
20 drops neroli or petitgrain essential oil

Pure neroli essential oil gives this cream its luxurious orange blossom scent, but less expensive alternatives include petit-grain, bergamot or ylang ylang oils.

Place the almond oil, olive or avocado oil and beeswax pieces in a ceramic bowl and put this inside a saucepan that has been half-filled with water. Gently heat on top of the stove until the beeswax has melted completely. Add the lecithin and beat the mixture vigorously.

Stir in the rosewater and remove from the heat. Add the essential oil of your choice to fragrance the cream.

Allow to cool slightly before pouring into a shallow tub or screw-top jar (scraping the cream from the sides of the mixing bowl before it sets). To use, massage liberally into rough, chapped skin on the hands, elbows and feet.

At home manicure

Equipment

Nail polish remover
Cotton wool pads
Nail scissors
Emery board or nail file
Cuticle cream (see recipe, page 140)
Rubber hoof stick
Orange sticks
Orange blossom massage cream (see recipe, page 141)

Wash hands and nails in warm, soapy water and dry thoroughly. Remove any nail polish with remover on cotton wool pads. Trim long nails with nail scissors and file into a smooth oval shape, using an emery board or non-metal nail file. Avoid 'sawing' backwards and forwards as this weakens the nail. The best way to file the nails is in one direction only.

After filing, rinse the fingertips in warm water and pat dry. Apply a small amount of *Cuticle cream* around each nail and massage into the cuticle and base of the nail. Leave for a few minutes for the cream to penetrate and soften the skin.

Next, take the rubber hoof stick and gently push back the cuticle from around each nail. Never force the skin back and avoid cutting or poking the cuticle as this can pierce the skin and lead to infections. When you have been around each cuticle, take an orange stick and wipe around the base of each nail to remove traces of cuticle cream.

Apply a generous dollop of *Orange blossom massage cream* and work into the fingers, palms and wrists. Each hand contains twenty-eight small bones and a complex network of muscles and tendons, so spend at least 10 minutes giving the hands a gentle massage. This not only releases tension and loosens up stiff joints but also increases blood circulation and keeps the skin feeling supple and smooth.

Aim to give the hands a manicure once a week, and in between treatments follow this seven-point plan to healthier hands.

- Always wear a pair of gloves or use a barrier cream when outside or doing chores such as gardening or the washing-up.
- Avoid plunging the hands into too-hot or freezing-cold water as this encourages dehydration and leads to skin chapping.
- Always use a sunblock when out in sunny weather to prevent the formation of brown 'age' spots on the backs of the hands.
- Get into the habit of using a rich hand cream last thing at night.
- Add a daily dose of cod liver oil or almond oil capsules to your diet to help strengthen weak nails.
- Always trim hang-nails to prevent them tearing or splitting.
- Avoid opening the mail, tins, jars etc. with the nails as this weakens the structure and encourages them to break off.

Hard-skin remover

50 g (2 oz) cocoa butter
50 g (2 oz) cornmeal (polenta)
25 g (1 oz) Fuller's earth
10 drops lemon or mandarin essential oil

This treatment is ideal for buffing away calluses that have formed on the hands or feet, or for smoothing pimply patches on elbows or knees.

In a small saucepan gently melt the cocoa butter. Remove from the heat and stir in the cornmeal and Fuller's earth until the mixture forms a thick paste. Beat in the essential oil to add a light fragrance.

To use, massage into areas of rough skin on the feet, hands, elbows and knees. Use firm, circular movements to help shift calluses and leave the skin feeling silky smooth. Wipe away excess cream with a warm, damp cloth or flannel. Follow with an application of *Orange blossom massage cream*.

At-home pedicure

Equipment

Nail polish remover
Cotton wool pads
Foot bath or washing-up bowl
Soap or *Soapwort cleanser* (see recipe, page 140)
Stiff nail brush
Small towel
Nail scissors
Emery board or nail file
Cuticle cream (see recipe, page 140)
Rubber hoof stick
Cuticle clippers
Orange blossom massage cream (see recipe, page 141)

First, remove any nail polish from the toenails with remover and cotton wool pads. Half-fill the footbath or washing-up bowl with warm water and soak the feet for at least 5 minutes to allow the skin to warm and soften.

Gently scrub the feet and toes with a stiff nail brush and soap or *Soapwort cleanser*. Dry the feet and toes thoroughly and trim long nails by cutting straight across with a small pair of nail scissors. Smooth any rough edges of the nails with an emery board or non-metal nail file.

Next, apply a small amount of *Cuticle cream* to each toenail and massage into the cuticles. Use a rubber hoof stick to gently encourage the cuticles away from the nail bed, but be careful not to jab or poke too vigorously as this can pierce the skin and lead to infections.

Use a sharp pair of cuticle clippers to cut away any small pieces of dead cuticle, but take care not to snip any living tissue. Spend the next ten minutes massaging the feet with a generous helping of *Orange blossom massage cream* – you will be rewarded for your efforts afterwards when your feet feel as though they are walking on air.

Finally, dust in between the toes with talcum powder (you can make your own by mixing together equal quantities of arrowroot and cornflour, scented with small pieces of chopped orange and lemon peel). Aim to give your feet a pedicure at least once a month to keep calluses, corns and bunions at bay.

In between treatments you can encourage healthy feet, ankles and toes by following these six steps to healthier feet.

- Switch heel heights during the day to give the feet and calves a break. If you wear high heels during the day, slip into a pair of pumps in the evening.
- Invest in a corrugated foot roller to give the feet a reflexology-style work-out during the day. Simply move the feet along the roller to stimulate the nerve endings on the soles of the feet.
- Use a rich moisture cream on your feet at night and wake up to softer toes.
- Always wear well-fitting shoes and have your feet professionally measured from time to time when choosing a new pair, in case of change.
- Apply a daily dab of *Cuticle cream* or almond oil to the toenails to keep cuticles soft and well conditioned.
- Always trim toenails straight across, never down at the sides, to prevent painful in-growing toenails.

Athletes foot bath

1 small onion, finely chopped
1 clove garlic, finely chopped
1 cm (½ in) fresh ginger root, finely grated
25 g (1 oz) fresh or dried sage
25 g (1 oz) fresh or dried rosemary
3.4 litres (6 pints) hot water
20 drops tea tree essential oil

This footbath treats fungal infections of the foot and is also invigorating for feet that are sore and tired from strenuous exercise such as running or skiing.

First, in a large saucepan, make a herbal infusion by adding the onion, garlic, ginger root and herbs to the hot water. Gently simmer for 5 minutes before removing from the heat and leaving to steep for 10 more minutes. Strain the liquid and allow to cool slightly.

Add the tea tree essential oil and pour the liquid into a footbath or washing-up bowl. Soak the feet in the warm water for 20 minutes, covering with a towel to prevent the heat from escaping.

Remove from the water and pat every part of the foot dry, especially in between the toes. Finish with a light dusting of medicated talcum powder or arrowroot that has been infused with the scent from a few whole juniper berries.

Hot oil smoother

50 ml (2 fl oz) almond oil
20 ml (4 tsp) wheatgerm oil
10 drops lavender essential oil
Pair of old cotton socks
Pair of cotton gloves

This is an excellent overnight intensive treatment for re-moisturising hard skin on the hands and feet. The hot oil rapidly soaks into the upper layers of skin and is sealed in with cotton socks and gloves. This encourages our natural body heat to boost penetration of the oil even further (cotton manicure gloves are available from major department stores and some chemists).

Warm the almond oil in a small saucepan. Add the wheatgerm oil and lavender essential oil and remove from the heat. Apply liberally to clean feet and hands, massaging well into the skin before covering with cotton socks and gloves. Leave overnight and in the morning the skin will feel fabulously soft and smooth.

Herbal Hair Care

Hair consists of a type of protein called keratin, which responds well to many beauty treatments. Keratin itself is a peculiar horny substance that also makes up our nails, and even the horns of wild animals. It is pushed out from hair follicles that cover the scalp and grows into long strands. Each hair strand has a central cortex which is soft and a coating of hard scales on the outside which are the cuticles. As with our skin, the hair is moisturised by the body's own protective oil called sebum. This is secreted from sebaceous glands in the scalp and travels along each hair strand to coat the cuticles, keeping them shiny and smooth. Unfortunately, many factors interfere with the health of our scalp and hair. Diet is important as the hair follicles rely on a steady stream of nutrients delivered daily by the blood supply.

The most important nutrients for healthy hair are Vitamins A, B-complex, C and D, together with zinc, iron and the essential fatty acids found mainly in vegetable oils. Other lifestyle factors that interfere with a healthy head of hair include smoking, excess alcohol, not taking enough exercise and too much stress. Our hormones also play an important part in the condition of our hair and can affect hair loss and scalp disorders such as dandruff. Most of the other problems that occur are inflicted by ourselves. Washing in harsh detergent-based shampoos, over-heating with hot hairdryers, curling tongs and heated rollers, or over-brushing and back-combing all conspire to reduce our hair to a mass of dry tangles.

The basic rules of effective hair care are simple and will dramatically improve the condition of all hair types.

- Wash hair gently in a mild shampoo. Vigorous scrubbing can stimulate the sebaceous glands to producing excess sebum and lead to greasy hair.
- Hair should be washed every other day or possibly once a day, if you live in a polluted, urban environment.
- Avoid using too much shampoo, which can strip away the scalp's naturally protective oils. One shampooing should be sufficient, unless your hair is full of styling products such as sticky lacquer or hair gel.
- All hair types will benefit from a light conditioner to protect the scales on the hair cuticle and encourage a glossy shine.
- Turn down the setting on your hairdryer to avoid over-heating the hair. This is especially important if your hair has been chemically treated with colourants or a perm. Ideally, let your hair dry naturally once in a while.
- Treat your hair to a weekly scalp massage which will encourage fresh blood supplies to flow to the surface of the scalp and feed the hair follicles.
- Dry and chemically damaged hair should be given an intensive moisturising treatment once a week.

Hair should be our crowning glory and it is easy to coax it into better condition with these herbal hair care recipes.

Sandalwood and soapwort shampoo

25 g (1 oz) chopped soapwort root
25 g (1 oz) dried chamomile flowers
250 ml (8 fl oz) hot water
20 drops sandalwood essential oil

This simple shampoo is gentle on the skin and suitable for all hair types.

Place the chopped soapwort root and chamomile flowers

in a bowl and pour on the almost-boiling water. Stir well, cover and leave overnight to infuse. In the morning, strain the liquid and add the drops of sandalwood essential oil.

To use, wet the hair and massage in a small amount of the mixture. Rinse and repeat if necessary. Although soapwort root is an efficient cleanser, it does not produce a lather like conventional detergent-based shampoos.

No-wash shampoo

50 g (2 oz) powdered orris root
25 g (1 oz) semolina or ground rice
10 drops lemon essential oil
10 drops neroli essential oil

This is a useful way of cleaning the hair when you can't or don't want to wash it with water. The method of dry-hair shampooing works best on short and medium-length hair and absorbs dirt, sebum and general grime from the hair and scalp.

In a large bowl mix the orris root and semolina or ground rice together. Sprinkle in the drops of essential oil and stir the mixture to distribute the fragrance. Transfer to a screw-top jar for storage.

To use, tip the head upside-down and brush the hair forward. Rub small amounts of the mixture into the scalp, starting at the base of the neck and working forward. Use a natural bristle brush to brush the hair thoroughly, working the mixture through the hair from the roots to the ends. Throw the head back and brush out any remaining particles of mixture. The hair will be left feeling clean, soft and fragrant.

Dry hair and scalp shampoo

25 g (1 oz) chopped soapwort root
500 ml (17 fl oz) hot water
25 g (1 oz) coconut oil
15 drops sandalwood or patchouli essential oil

This shampoo gently re-moisturises the hair and scalp.

Add the chopped soapwort root to the hot water, cover and leave to infuse overnight. In the morning, remove the pieces of root and strain the liquid. In a small saucepan, gently melt the coconut oil and add to the soapwort decoction.

Stir in the drops of essential oil to subtly fragrance the shampoo. To use, massage a small amount of the pre-warmed mixture into the scalp and rinse with plenty of hot water. Note that the soapwort root has excellent cleansing properties but does not produce much lather. This shampoo is mild enough to be used on children and babies, but use chamomile essential oil for the fragrance as this is gentler on their scalps.

Cleansing clay shampoo

100 g (4 oz) Fuller's earth
100 g (4 oz) coconut oil
120 ml (4 fl oz) chamomile tea
30 ml (2 tbsp) cider vinegar
10 drops peppermint essential oil

This unusual shampoo is especially good for removing flakes of dead skin from the scalp and for absorbing excess sebum. The peppermint oil also makes the shampoo feel refreshing on the skin and boosts the blood to the scalp.

Place the coconut oil in a small bowl and stir in the Fuller's earth powder. Set to one side while you make the chamomile tea by infusing 1 dessertspoonful (10 ml) of dried chamomile flowers, or 1 chamomile herb tea bag, in a cupful of almost-boiling water. Leave to steep for 5 minutes before straining.

Beat in the chamomile tea and cider vinegar and transfer to a large, shallow tub or jar.

To use, rub small amounts of the mixture into the scalp, massaging gently to dislodge dead skin cells. Leave for 5 minutes before rinsing thoroughly with plenty of warm water. As this cleansing treatment removes excess oil from the scalp and hair shafts it should be followed with a light conditioner.

Natural hair rinses

Herbal hair rinses are a
poo. Based on natura
correct pH balance to
remove the mineral de
washing, and encourag

- *Normal hair*. Fresh eld
  Simmer with water f
  the juice. Apply to t
  minutes then shamp
  vinegar added to yo
  way to restore the c
  gleaming.
- *Dry and chemically pr*
  by hard water so mak
  5 ml (1 tsp) domestic borax in 3.4 litres (6 pints) of warm
  water. You may also add 5 ml (1 tsp) cider vinegar to restore pH balance, and 6 drops chamomile essential oil to
  fragrance the hair.
- *Oily hair*. Make a herbal infusion based on 15 ml (1 tbsp)
  freshly chopped mint leaves, 15 ml (1 tbsp) freshly chopped
  rosemary leaves, and the juice of 1 lemon mixed in 300 ml
  (½ pint) hot water. Leave to infuse for 15 minutes, strain
  and use as a final hair rinse.
- *Lank or limp hair*. Make a herbal infusion of 15 ml (1 tbsp)
  fresh chopped rosemary leaves in 250 ml (8 fl oz) hot water.
  Leave to steep for 15 minutes, strain and add the juice of 1
  lemon and 30 ml (2 tbsp) flat beer. Mix well and apply to
  the hair as a final rinse after shampooing.
- *Blonde hair*. Use the freshly squeezed juice of two lemons
  mixed with an equal quantity of water. Comb through wet
  hair after shampooing and leave for 15–20 minutes before
  rinsing. Alternatively, add 100 g (4 oz) dried chamomile
  flowers to 500 ml (17 fl oz) almost-boiling water. Leave to
  infuse for 30 minutes and use as a final rinse to bring out
  naturally blonde highlights in the hair.
- *Dark hair*. Make an infusion based on 25 g (1 oz) sage leaves
  in 3.4 litres (6 pints) of almost-boiling water. Steep for 2
  hours. Leave on the hair for 30 minutes before rinsing out.
  Alternatively, mix 1 cup of strong black coffee with the

freshly squeezed juice of one lemon. Leave on the hair for 30 minutes after shampooing before rinsing out.

- *Red hair*. Save the cooking water from beetroots to use as a natural plum-coloured hair dye. Use sparingly and cover the hands with rubber gloves or you will end up with purple fingers, too! Alternatively, use a glass of red wine as a final rinse after shampooing to bring out naturally auburn highlights in the hair.

Intensive hair conditioner

15 ml (1 tbsp) black strap molasses
2 egg yolks
50 ml (2 fl oz) avocado or almond oil

This unconventional hair conditioner works well on dry, chemically processed hair as it leaves the hair strands unusually shiny and smooth.

In a small bowl, vigorously beat together the black strap molasses and egg yolks until they form a stiff paste. Add the avocado or almond oil and mix again.

Apply to dry hair, working through the ends of the hair up towards the roots. Leave for 15–20 minutes and wash the hair as usual, using two applications of shampoo to remove all traces of the conditioner.

Sesame sun-screener

50 ml (2 fl oz) sesame oil
25 g (1 oz) coconut oil
10 ml (2 tsp) wheatgerm oil

The sesame oil in this formula shields the hair from about a third of the sun's damaging ultra-violet rays. This emollient hair sunscreen also acts as an intensive conditioner and prevents the hair from drying out in the sun. It is especially good for dry, tinted or permed hair, which is more porous than most and therefore prone to sun damage.

Place the sesame oil and coconut oil in a small saucepan and heat gently until the coconut oil has melted. Remove from the heat and stir in the wheatgerm oil. Pour into a small bottle or jar and shake well before use.

Apply by combing through dry hair just before you go out sun-bathing.

Hot-oil hair restructuriser

50 ml (2 fl oz) olive oil
10 drops sandalwood essential oil

This treatment is especially good for dry, tinted or permed hair which has become brittle and unmanageable.

Gently warm the olive oil in a small saucepan. Add the drops of essential oil and stir thoroughly. Apply to dry hair and comb through from the roots to the ends using a wide-toothed comb. Massage any remaining oil gently into the scalp.

Wrap the hair and scalp in a towel, turban-style, to seal in the body heat from the scalp. Leave for 20 minutes before shampooing twice with a mild shampoo.

Aromatic pomade

50 ml (2 fl oz) almond oil
25 ml (1 fl oz) castor oil
20 drops neroli essential oil
10 drops lavender essential oil
10 drops lemon essential oil

This natural hair shiner is based on a Renaissance recipe, when fragrant oils were popular among noblemen and women to keep their hair smelling sweet.

In a screw-top bottle or jar, mix together the almond and castor oils. Add the aromatic essential oils and shake well. To use, apply a few drops to the fingertips and massage into the hair. Alternatively, rub a few drops on to the bristles of a hairbrush and brush through the hair. This wonderfully fragrant mixture leaves the hair subtly scented, and with a healthy, glossy shine.

Styling lotion

250 ml (8 fl oz) boiling water
50 g (2 oz) sugar
30 ml (2 tbsp) flat beer
15 drops lemon or neroli essential oil

This traditional hair-styling lotion was popular during the war years when conventional setting lotions were not so readily available.

Dissolve the sugar in the boiling water and leave to cool. Add the flat beer and essential oil (this is important to avoid smelling like a brewery). Apply to wet or damp hair after shampooing and use to set the hair on rollers or with curling tongs. Left-over liquid can be kept in a plastic spray bottle and used in between washes when re-styling the hair.

Dry-ends cream

50 g (2 oz) coconut oil
50 g (2 oz) cocoa butter
30 ml (2 tbsp) almond oil
15 drops neroli essential oil

Although nothing mends split-ends once they have broken, this mixture temporarily seals them and discourages the hair shaft from splitting further.

In a small saucepan melt together the coconut oil with the cocoa butter. Remove from the heat and stir in the almond oil. When the mixture has cooled slightly add the neroli essential oil.

To use, rub a small amount between the fingertips and apply sparingly to dry hair ends in between washes. This mixture may also be used as an intensive hair-conditioning treatment before shampooing. Simply massage into the hair and scalp, cover the head with a towel to seal in body heat and leave for 20 minutes before shampooing out.

Re-moisturising scalp lotion

50 ml (2 fl oz) avocado oil
50 ml (2 fl oz) almond oil
25 ml (1 fl oz) cider vinegar
30 ml (2 tbsp) strong nettle tea
10 drops peppermint essential oil
10 drops lavender essential oil

A good treatment for itchy, flaky scalps, or for those prone to thinning hair.

Measure the avocado and almond oils into a screw-top bottle or jar. Add the cider vinegar and shake well. Make the strong nettle tea by infusing 1 dessertspoonful (10 ml) of dried or fresh nettle leaves in ½ cup of almost-boiling water. Leave to steep for 10 minutes, strain and add the liquid to the oil and vinegar mixture.

Shake vigorously to emulsify the liquid and when cool, add the drops of peppermint and lavender essential oils.

To use, shake the bottle and rub a small amount daily into the scalp by parting the hair and applying with cotton wool.

Cradle cap treatment

50 ml (2 fl oz) almond oil
50 ml (2 fl oz) calendula oil
10 drops chamomile essential oil

Cradle cap is a common scalp complaint during infancy and is easy to improve with this gentle treatment. Both the almond and calendula oils are extremely soothing on a baby's fragile scalp.

Mix together the almond and calendula oils and add the chamomile essential oil. Store the mixture in a screw-top bottle or jar and shake vigorously before use.

To use, massage a small amount of the mixture into the affected area before bathing. Lightly shampoo using a mild, baby shampoo and pat the scalp dry. For severe cases, a few drops of the massage oil may be rubbed into the affected area in between hair washes.

Anti-dandruff hair tonic

1.2 litres (2 pints) strong nettle tea
250 ml (8 fl oz) birch infusion

While it is usual for the scalp to shed dead skin cells, dandruff is a scalp condition that occurs when the surface skin cells grow faster than normal, resulting in a build-up of scurf on the scalp. Dry, itching scalps may be caused by an allergic reaction to your shampoo, or simply by the scalp drying out. Drinking plenty of water and sipping burdock tea may help. Investing in a small humidifier for your home or office may also be useful. Nettles contain many beneficial minerals, including iron and zinc, and both nettles and birch have been used by herbalists since Roman times to treat scalp disorders.

To make the tonic, simmer a handful of young nettle tops in 1.2 litres (2 pints) water for 2 hours. Alternatively, make a strong nettle tea using 4 dessertspoonfuls (40 ml) of dried nettle leaves or 4 nettle herb tea bags. While the nettle tea is infusing, make the birch infusion by stirring 15 ml (1 tbsp) fresh or dried birch leaves into a cupful of almost-boiling water. Leave to steep for 30 minutes. When the two infusions are ready, mix together and pour into bottles. Apply to the hair and scalp 2–3 times a week, or use as a final hair rinse after washing (do not rinse out).

Anti-itch scalp rinse

500 ml (17 fl oz) nettle tea
30 ml (2 tbsp) cider vinegar
6 drops chamomile essential oil

This is a useful final hair rinse to soothe dry, flaky scalps.

Make the nettle tea by infusing 50 g (2 oz) of fresh, young nettle tops in 500 ml (17 fl oz) of almost-boiling water. Alternatively, use 2 dessertspoonfuls (20 ml) of dried nettles or 2 nettle herb tea bags. Allow to steep for 10 minutes before straining the infusion. Add the cider vinegar and chamomile essential oil and stir well. Pour over the scalp after the final rinse and massage gently into the skin. Do not rinse out. Repeat three times a week.

RECIPE MEASUREMENTS

Liquid measures

Metric	Imperial
2.5 ml	½ teaspoon
5 ml	1 teaspoon
10 ml	1 dessertspoon
15 ml	1 tablespoon or ½ fl oz
20 ml	¾ fl oz
25 ml	1 fl oz
50 ml	2 fl oz
100 ml	3½ fl oz
120 ml	4 fl oz
150 ml	5 fl oz or ¼ pint
175 ml	6 fl oz
200 ml	7 fl oz or ⅓ pint
250 ml	8 fl oz
275 ml	9 fl oz
300 ml	10 fl oz or ½ pint
350 ml	12 fl oz
450 ml	15 fl oz or ¾ pint
600 ml	20 fl oz or 1 pint
750 ml	1¼ pints
1 litre	1¾ pints

Solid measures

Metric	Imperial
10 g	¼ oz
15 g	½ oz
20 g	¾ oz
25 g	1 oz
50 g	2 oz
100 g	4 oz or ¼ lb
225 g	8 oz or ½ lb
350 g	12 oz or ¾ lb
450 g	16 oz or 1 lb

ESSENTIAL OILS GUIDE

Name	Principal properties
Basil	Mentally stimulating
Bayleaf	Uplifting
Cedarwood	Diuretic, toning
Chamomile	Soothing, calming, naturally antibiotic
Clary sage	Balancing, restoring, uplifting
Cypress	Toning, diuretic
Eucalyptus	Invigorating, anti-inflammatory, antibiotic
Frankincense	Uplifting, meditative, purifying
Geranium	Soothing, toning, strengthening
Hyssop	Naturally antibiotic, warming, comforting
Jasmine	Uplifting, energising, aphrodisiac
Juniper berry	Anti-fungal, diuretic, stimulating
Lavender	Balancing, antibiotic/viral/fungal, toning
Lemon	Diuretic, stimulating, refreshing
Mandarin	Refreshing, toning, fortifying
Marjoram	Calming, sedating
Melissa	Balancing, uplifting, refreshing
Myrrh	Anti-fungal, anti-inflammatory
Neroli	Uplifting, restoring, fortifying
Patchouli	Anti-fungal, strengthening, calming
Peppermint	Invigorating, refreshing, relaxing
Petitgrain	Calming, strengthening, relaxing
Pine	Stimulating, strengthening
Rose	Soothing, strengthening, relaxing
Rosemary	Diuretic, strengthening, invigorating
Sage	Anti-fungal, strengthening, stimulating
Sandalwood	Uplifting, comforting, aphrodisiac, soothing
Tea tree	Antibiotic/viral/fungal, cleansing
Thyme	Antibiotic/viral/fungal, stimulating
Ylang ylang	Invigorating, refreshing, aphrodisiac

All essential oils are also highly antiseptic. Consult a trained aromatherapist if using essential oils to treat medical conditions, or if using during pregnancy.

Glossary

Anti-inflammatory – a substance that reduces inflammation of the tissues, so reducing pain and swelling. Some anti-inflammatory plant extracts contain substances that are similar to steroids, such as marigold and licorice. Others contain painkilling ingredients similar to aspirin; for example, Balm of Gilead and willowbark (from which aspirin was first extracted). Anti-inflammatory plants, such as dandelion, citrus oils and marigold, may also work by stimulating the circulation.

Anti-oxidant – a substance that prevents the formation of destructive free radicals within the body and skin. Natural anti-oxidants include Vitamins C and E and beta-carotene, which also act as preservatives in skincare recipes.

Antiseptic – many plants have antiseptic properties, meaning they fight infections and germs on the surface of the skin. Most essential oils are antiseptic and plants containing high levels of tannins are also antiseptic. Others, such as marigold, thyme and tea tree, also have anti-fungal effects.

Anti-spasmodic – a term given to herbs or other substances that prevent or relieve spasms within the body.

Aromatherapy – the therapeutic use of essential oils to treat many kinds of disorders, notably skin complaints, cellulite, hormonal problems and stress.

Astringent – any substance that causes the contraction of body tissue. In skincare it is a term given to liquids that temporarily tighten the skin. In herbalism, plants with astringent properties work by binding protein molecules together to provide a protective surface on delicate areas such as mucous membranes, to prevent inflammation and aid healing. Astringent plants tend to have a high tannin content.

Carrier oils – the vegetable oils used in aromatherapy to carry the more concentrated essential oils on to the skin. Common carrier oils include almond and grapeseed oils.

Decoction – a term used by herbalists for a liquid made by pouring cold water on to finely chopped plant material and simmering. Used when extracting the active ingredients from tough types of ingredients, such as bark and roots, which are difficult to infuse. Decoctions can be made by simmering the plant material at just below boiling point for 6–8 hours, straining, squeezing and storing in the fridge for up to three days (see also **Tincture**). Decoctions may also be bought readymade from herbal suppliers.

Demulcent – a term given to plant extracts that have naturally soothing effects on the surface of the skin.

Diuretic – a substance that increases the flow of urine and reduces puffiness due to fluid retention in the tissues.

Eczema – an increasingly common and frequently distressing skin condition most common during childhood and puberty. Characterised by patches of itching, scaling skin that may produce a clear discharge if scratched. Sometimes triggered by allergies to groups of foods such as dairy products, wheat-based foods and citrus fruits. Also linked to other allergic conditions such as asthma and psoriasis.

Emollient – a term used to describe a substance that smooths and lubricates the surface of the skin.

Essential oils – the fragrant, volatile and highly concentrated essences extracted from leaves, flowers, roots and bark of plants. The term 'essential' refers to the fact that they are essences.

Expectorant – a remedy that encourages the production of mucus and bronchial secretions in the respiratory passages in order to clear airways.

Extract – a substance made by placing pieces of a plant or herb in water, alcohol or a solvent in order to remove its active ingredients. Once these have been removed from the plant or herb, the liquid may be evaporated off, leaving behind the pure extract.

Free radicals – the principal cause of skin ageing and most degenerative diseases within the human body. Caused when highly active and destructive chemical compounds from oxygen are produced by oxidation. Processes that trigger the production of free radicals include ultra-violet radiation from the sun and air-borne chemical pollutants.

Homoeopathy – a form of holistic medicine which is both safe and effective in treating numerous medical conditions. Based on the idea of helping the body to heal itself by providing traces of potentially toxic substances that trigger the body's own immune response.

Hormones – substances created within the body by various glands, e.g., adrenalin from the adrenal glands, and thyroxin from the thyroid gland. Used to regulate numerous bodily functions, including emotions.

Impetigo – a highly infectious skin disease common in childhood. Recognised by blisters on the face that dry to leave a yellowish crust. Best treated with a vitamin-enriched diet and antiseptic remedies.

Infusion – a preparation made by steeping a plant or herb in water to extract its active ingredients. An infusion is made by pouring boiling water over finely chopped plant material, such as leaves or dried flowers. Herb teas are simply an infusion of dried flowers, leaves, etc. Most parts of the plant are suitable for creating infusions, including ground stalks and powdered roots (see also **Decoction**). The infusion should be made by pouring boiling water on to the plant material and leaving to soak for up to 1 hour. Liquids should then be refrigerated and will last several days.

Inhalations – Many of the active ingredients in substances such as essential oils are carried through their smell. One way to make use of these is with an inhalation which carries the volatile components of the oil into the brain cells located at the top of the nose. The smelliest herbs which have the highest content of volatile oils are the most suitable for inhalations, e.g., thyme, rosemary, lavender and eucalyptus.

Lotion – a light-weight, non-greasy cream that tends to be used on larger areas of skin; e.g., body lotions. A lotion may also be made from herbal infusions and applied to the skin with cotton wool.

Lymphatic system – a network of vessels or lymph channels that parallels the blood circulatory system. Lymph itself is a milky fluid that circulates around the body picking up debris and unwanted toxins from cells. Unlike the blood supply, the lymphatic system does not have the heart to pump it around the body and so relies on massage and exercise to keep it moving.

Medical herbalism – a traditional form of medicine practised by those who have undergone lengthy professional training, recognised by the Medicines Act of 1968. Practitioners treat the patient as a whole and use herbal remedies to cure the long-term cause of the problem, not only its individual symptoms. The minimum length of training is four years, although many medical herbalists train for longer, and study other healing arts such as acupuncture and iridology.

Mucilages – substances containing complex carbohydrates that give some plants a slimy quality. Used in cosmetic preparations to make natural gels or to thicken liquids and creams; e.g. carrageen moss. They are not absorbed by the body and pass through the system if swallowed, making useful bulking agents and laxatives; e.g., linseeds.

Oxidation – a process where a substance is chemically combined with oxygen and its original structure altered or destroyed. When skin creams 'oxidise', their oils and fat are affected by the oxygen in the atmosphere and they turn rancid.

Phytotherapy – a European term given to the use of plant remedies. In France, phytotherapy is a recognised part of medicine and is included in hospital training. Phytotherapy uses more traditional remedies, based on herbal extracts and essential oils.

Poultice – a heated pack that can be applied directly to the skin to relieve pain, swelling or tenderness in the joints or muscles. Made by mixing herbal infusions or chopped pieces of plant with hot water and applying on cotton muslin or a flannel. An effective method to draw the pus from pimples and boils, or splinters from under the skin (use sterile gauze on open wounds).

Psoriasis – a severe skin disorder associated with allergic problems such as asthma and eczema. Characterised by inflamed, red, scaling skin and notoriously hard to treat. Many herbalists report good results by dietary and lifestyle changes, combined with detoxifying herbal remedies; it is aggravated by stress, alcohol and a refined food diet. Topical applications of soothing herbal extras such as calendula may also help.

Resins – the gummy secretions from tree bark that melt when heated. Mostly insoluble in water so need to be used in an alcohol solution. Resins contain many powerful healing agents and are highly antiseptic; e.g., Balm of Gilead and myrrh.

Stimulant – any substance used to increase the power of the body to boost strength and energy.

Tannins – substances found in plant leaves and bark containing natural phenols. They have astringent qualities and are useful in skincare to tone and protect the skin.

Tincture – similar to a decoction or an infusion, but in this case the plant liquid is made by steeping in a mixture of alcohol and water. They are especially suitable for plants that have a high content of resins or essential oils. Because of their alcohol content, tinctures have a longer shelf-life and are more readily available in a highly concentrated form. Most herbal tinctures contain approximately thirty-five per cent alcohol.

Tonic – any substance that promotes energy and well-being. In skincare the term is used for liquids that tone the skin and encourage an increased blood supply to surface skin tissues. Herbalists also use plant extracts as internal tonics to pep up the system and strengthen the skin from within. Most plant-based skincare recipes have a tonic effect on the skin.

Further Information

Herbs

Medical Herbalism

When choosing a medical herbalist, always look for the letters of qualification after their names, MNIMH or FNIMH. These guarantee that you are in safe, trained and caring hands. To find your nearest qualified medical herbalist contact the Hon. General Secretary, The National Institute of Medical Herbalists, 41, Hatherley Road, Winchester, Hampshire SO22 6RR. Please enclose a large, stamped, self-addressed envelope for a register of practitioners.

The Herb Society
PO Box 599, London SW11 4RW
Annual membership currently costs £14 (concessions £10). Membership includes two copies of *Herbs*, the only specialist magazine devoted to all aspects of herbs, and four copies of *Herbarium* each year. Members also receive discounts from numerous herbal suppliers.

Herbal Suppliers

G. Baldwin & Co.
171–173, Walworth Road, London SE17 1RW
(071-703 5550)
Medical herbalists who stock a wide range of herbal powders and accessories. Mail-order available.

Barwinnock Herbs
Barrhill, Ayrshire, KA26 ORB
(0465 82338)
Wide variety of medicinal and culinary herbs, including organically grown varieties. Many variegated and unusually perfumed varieties. Also herb-drying cabinets. Mail-order available.

Blackbrook Herb Gardens
Blackbrook Cottage, Alderley Road, Wilmslow, Cheshire SK9 1PZ
(0625 539166)
Specialist herb plants by post. Free catalogue.

Brin School Fields
The Old School, Flichity, Inverness IV1 2XD
(0808 3288)
Herb plants, toiletries and demonstrations. Mail-order available.

Caroline Holmes Herbs
Denham End Farm, Denham, Bury St Edmunds, Suffolk IP29 5EE
(0284 810653)
Large variety of fresh and dried herbs. Also day courses, lectures and talks. Mail-order available.

Churchfield Herbs
2, High Street, Yardley Gobion, Towcester, Northants NN12 7UB
(0908 543276)
Fresh and dried herbs and wild flowers, spices and essential oils. Mail-order available.

Culpeper
Hadstock Road, Linton, Cambridge, CB1 6NJ
(0223 891196)
This is the mail-order department, which supplies a wide range of dried herbs, herbal ingredients and essential oils by post. Culpeper also have several retail outlets, including London, Cambridge and Bath.

Dolma
19 Royce Avenue, Hucknall, Notts NG15 6FU
(0602 634237)
Supply herbal toiletries and ingredients, including essential oils and vegetable oils. Mail-order available.

Heaven Scent Herbs
Rose Cottage, Heathfield, Langford Budville, Nr Wellington, Somerset TA21 ORO
(0823 400689)
Supply dried herbs and essential oils. Mail-order available.

Herb and Goat Farm
Waterlane, Selsey, Stroud, Glos GL5 5LW
(0453 766632)
Herb gardens and shop. Supply fresh and dried herbs. Mail-order available.
Also Selsey Herb Shop branches at 22 Castle Street, Cirencester, and 4 George Street, Nailsworth, Gloucestershire.

Herb and Heather Centre
West Haddlesey, Nr Selby, North Yorkshire Y08 8QA
(0757 228279)
Herb consultants, seminars and courses. Wide range available by mail-order, including organically grown varieties.

Iden Croft Herbs
Frittenden Road, Staplehurst, Kent TN12 ODN
(0580 891432)
Large herb garden for the blind and disabled. Shop selling fresh and dried herbs. Mail-order available.

Magic Garden Herbs
18 Spillman's Road, Rodborough, Stroud, Gloucestershire
Organic, lunar-grown herb plants and seeds. Mail-order only.

Neals Yard
15 Neals Yard, Covent Garden, London WC2H 9DP
(071-379 7222) Mail-order available on 0865 245436
Extensive range of medicinal herbs, including dried herbs, powders and herbal tinctures. Organically grown varieties available. Also essential oils, vegetable oils and cosmetic-making ingredients. Smaller branch at Chelsea Farmers' Market, and the Glades shopping centre in Bromley.

Pepper Alley Herbs
The Spice Warehouse, Pepper Alley, Banbury, Oxon OX16 8JB
(0295 253888)
Large range of culinary and medicinal herbs and spices. Also essential and floral oils. Mail-order available.

Salley Gardens
8 Radcliffe Mount, West Bridgford, Nottingham NG2 5FY
(0602 813690)
Rare medicinal and wildflower plants and seeds. Mail-order available.

Samares Herbs a Plenty
Samares Manor, St Clement, Jersey, Channel Islands
(0534 79635)
Herb shop and gardens. Talks from April to October.

Aromatherapy Practitioners and Training

The International Federation of Aromatherapists (IFA)
The Department of Continuing Education, Royal Masonic Hospital,
Ravenscourt Park, London W6 OTN
Send an SAE for a list of local, accredited practitioners and aroma-
therapy training courses. The IFA also publish a regular newsletter
which gives details of suppliers of high-quality essential oils.

The International Society of Professional Aromatherapists
41, Leicester Road, Hinckley, Leicestershire LE10 1LW
Send an SAE for a list of their qualified aromatherapist members.

Aromatherapy Associates
68, The Maltings, Fulmead Street, London SW6 2BY
(071-731 8129)
Supply excellent ready-made blends of essential oils, electric oil
burners and offer training courses. Also run a treatment clinic.
Mail-order available.

Eve Taylor Institute of Clincal Aromatherapy
22, Bromley Road, London SE6 2TP
(081-690 2149)
Aromatherapy courses and supplier of essential oils. Mail-order
available.

The Association of Tisserand Aromatherapists
PO Box 746, Hove BN3 3XA
Send an SAE for details of aromatherapy courses under the direc-
tion of Robert Tisserand.

London School of Aromatherapy
PO Box 780, London NW5 1DY
Send a large SAE for details of training courses and a list of their
trained aromatherapists country-wide.

Shirley Price Aromatherapy
PO Box 29, Hinckley, Leicestershire LE10 OFT
(0455 615466)
Extensive aromatherapy training courses, seminars, books and
videos. Also suppliers of high-quality essential oils and carrier oils.
Mail-order available.

Essential Oil Suppliers

Aladdin Aromas
Fellview, Nenthead, Alston, Cumbria CA9 3PS
(0434 381919)
Suppliers of essential oils, absolutes and carrier oils. Member of the
Natural Medicines Society. Mail-order available.

Aqua Oleum
The Old Convent, Beeches Green, Stroud, Glos GL5 4AD
(0453 753555)
Suppliers of essential oils, cold-pressed carrier oils. Mail-order
available.

Bay House Aromatics
296a, Ditchling Road, Brighton, Sussex BN1 6JG
(0273 559444)
Suppliers of essential oils, carrier oils, dispensing bottles, pipettes
and aromatherapy books. Mail-order available.

Bodytreats
15, Approach Road, London SW20 8BA
(081-543 7633)
Suppliers of organic essential oils and quality carrier oils. Mail-
order available.

Essentially Oils
Blacksmiths Hill, Aynho, Banbury, Oxon OX17 3AH
(0869 811108)
Suppliers of essential oils and aromatherapy skincare products.

Fleur
8, Baden Road, London N8 7RJ
(081-340 4097)
Suppliers of organic essential oils, cold-pressed carrier oils, amber
bottles and storage cases. Mail-order available.

Lothian Herbs
1, Peffermill Industrial Estate, Peffermill Road, Edinburgh EH16
5UY
(031-661 9803)
Wide selection of essential oils, carrier oils, floral waters and aromatherapy books. Mail-order available.

Meadows
Forest Farmhouse, Pope Street, Godmersham, Canterbury, Kent
CT4 7DN
(0227 731489)
Suppliers of essential oils, cold-pressed carrier oils and vaporisers.
Mail-order available.

Quintessence
3a, Birch Avenue, Whitwick, Leicester LE67 5GB
(0530 838358)
Suppliers of essential oils, absolutes, cold-pressed vegetable oils, amber glass and PVC bottles.

Homoeopathic Information

There are general practitioners in many parts of the country who provide homoeopathic treatment – either privately or within the National Health Service – for skin disorders. Names and addresses of GPs in different areas can be provided by the Homoeopathic Trust, Hahnemann House, 2, Powis Place, Great Ormond Street, London WC1N 3HT. Telephone 071-837 9469.

For details of non-medically qualified homoeopaths contact The Society of Homoeopaths, 47 Canada Grove, Bognor Regis, West Sussex, PO21 1DW. Telephone 0243 860678.

Homoeopathic Suppliers

The following homoeopathic pharmacies also have a mail-order service:
Ainsworths
38, New Cavendish Street, London W1M 7LH
(071-935 5330)

Ainsworths
40–44, High Street, Caterham, Surrey CR3 5UB
(0883 340332)

Buxton and Grant
176, Whiteladies Road, Bristol BS8 2XU
(0272 735025)

Galen Pharmacy
1, South Terrace, South Street, Dorchester, Dorset DT1 1DE
(0305 63996)

Goulds
14, Crowndale Road, London NW1 1TT
(071-388 4752)

Nelson's Pharmacy
73, Duke Street, London W1M 6BY
(071-629 3118)

Weleda
Heanor Road, Ilkeston, Derbyshire DE7 8DR
(0602 303151)

Miscellaneous

John Bell and Croydon
52-54, Wigmore Street, London W1H OAU
(071-935 5555)
Stock a wide range of herbal supplements and sundries, pharmacy
items, waxes, oils and accessories, such as body brushes. Mail-
order available.

Green Farm Nutrition Centre
Burwash Common, East Sussex TN19 7LX
(0435 882482)
Supply natural bristle body brushes as well as a wide range of herbal and nutritional supplements. Mail-order available.

Molton Brown
5 Iron Bridge House, 3 Bridge Approach, London NW1 8BD
(071-911 0070)
Supply natural bristle body brushes, loofah mitts, manicure equipment, etc., as well as a wide range of natural-based toiletries and
cosmetics. Mail-order available.

USEFUL ADDRESSES

Action Against Allergy
24–26, High Street, Hampton Hill, Middlesex TW12 1PD

Acne Support Group
16 Dufours Place, Broadwick Street, London W1V 1FE

British Register of Complementary Medicine
Institute of Complementary Medicine, PO Box 194, London SE16
1QZ
(071-237 5165)

Disfigurement Guidance Centre
PO Box 7, Cupar, Fife, Scotland KY15 4PF
(0333 312350)

Evening Primrose Oil Office
4 Cupar Road, London SW11 4JW
Offers free help and guidance to the public.

National Eczema Society
Tavistock House North, Tavistock Square, London WC1H 9RS
(071-388 4097)

The Natural Medicines Society
Edith Lewis House, Ilkeston, Derbyshire DE7 8EJ

Psoriasis Association
7 Milton Street, Northampton NN2 7JG
(0604 711129)

Please send an SAE when contacting any of the above organisations

FURTHER READING

If you have enjoyed *Liz Earle's Natural Beauty*, you may also be interested in two other titles by Liz Earle, also published by Vermilion. *Vital Oils* contains a wealth of personal and scientific evidence regarding the effect of oils both on the skin and within the body. *Vital Oils* also contains valuable dietary advice about supplements, such as evening primrose oil and cod liver oil, as well as information for those with PMT, skin disorders and arthritis. In addition, *Vital Oils* gives a complete guide to aromatherapy and practical information about essential oils.

Save Your Skin with Vital Oils is also essential reading for those interested in preserving their looks. This book contains a step-by-step guide to facial exercises and massage that will wipe years off your looks. It also includes delicious recipes to literally feed your face.

Both *Vital Oils* and *Save Your Skin with Vital Oils* by Liz Earle are available from bookshops or by mail-order from Murlyn Services on 0279 427203 (order are dispatched within twenty-four hours and are sent postage and packing free).

Index